S0-AAA-860

Volleyball Today

Volleyball Today

Marv Dunphy
Head Coach, Men's Volleyball Program
Pepperdine University, CA

Rod Wilde
Member, United States Men's National Volleyball Team

Series Editor for West's Physical Activities Series

Robert J. O'Connor, Ed.D.
Los Angeles Pierce College

West Publishing Company
St. Paul   New York   Los Angeles   San Francisco

Cover Photo:	David Hanover
Text Photos:	David Hanover Photography
Additional Photos:	U.S. National Team Photos, Pepperdine Athletic Department
Composition:	Patti Zeman
Production:	Miyake Illustration & Design

COPYRIGHT © 1991 by   WEST PUBLISHING COMPANY
610 Opperman Drive
P.O. Box 64526
St. Paul, MN 55164–0526

All rights reserved

Printed in the United States of America

98 97 96 95 94 93 92   8 7 6 5 4 3 2 1

Library of Congress Cataloging-in-Publication Data

Dunphy, Marv
  Volleyball Today/Marv Dunphy, Rod Wilde.
  p. cm.—(West's physical activities series)
  Includes bibliographical references and index.
  ISBN 0-314-83711-6
  1. Volleyball—United States I. Wilde, Rod, II. Title, III. Series.
  GV1015.55.086   1991
  796.325'0973—dc20
                                                       91-8097
                                                       CIP

Table of Contents

Preface

It is the fervent hope of the authors that this book will present an approach to learning the game of volleyball that will rapidly take the learner from basic beginner play to the intermediate or advanced levels. The quicker the player gets to the high level of play, the greater his or her enjoyment of the game.

The authors have attempted to explain the techniques and strategies that they teach in their beginning, intermediate, and advanced classes and in their instructional camps. To some people it may seem that there is more than beginning-level skill presented herein. Since every student learns at a different pace, there may be too much for some and not enough for others. For that reason we have presented in each fundamental chapter a checklist for progression of learning.

The fundamentals and team play of volleyball have rapidly evolved, as has the method of teaching. The older "part to whole" progression has been proven much less effective than the "whole" skill methodology.

Additionally, the pedagogy of teaching skills has been found to be much more effective in a game-related situation than in non-game-related drills.

Acknowledgments

The development of this text could not have progressed without the helpful criticisms and suggestions from colleagues. The authors gratefully acknowledge the following:

Patti Barrett,
Southwest Texas State University

Ed Bigham
Southern Illinois University

Dave Markland
University of North Carolina

Elaine Michaelis
Brigham Young University

Eldin Onsgard
Los Angeles Pierce College

Tom Peterson
Pennsylvania State University

Additionally, the authors would like to thank the players Glenn Sato, Nina Mathies, Rick McLaughlin and Elaine Roque who served as models for the text photographs, and David Hanover for his excellent photography. Special thanks goes to the staff of West Publishing Company—specifically to Theresa O'Dell for her excellent editorial advice and support, and Mario Rodriguez for his meticulous scrutiny in the production of this text.

Now, learn—play—and enjoy the game of volleyball!

Foreword

Marv Dunphy is an outstanding teacher. This statement has been earned and proven by directing gold medal success at both collegiate and Olympic levels. Success in team sports is always the result of the players being taught the ability to properly and quickly execute the individual fundamentals and channel their abilities into the team concept. Coach Dunphy has shown an ability to do this second to none. Every coach and every player can greatly enhance their ability by carefully studying the techniques explained in this book.

Coach John Wooden
10-time NCAA National Champion Coach

Volleyball Today offers the combined talents of two technical experts in the sport. Their treatment of each volleyball skill is unparalled. The sequence of detailed explanations, checklist, common error and drills with diagrams provides the reader with complete coverage of all aspects of each volleyball skill. Thus, the sequence captures the skill for the beginner, intermediate and advanced player, as well as for the teacher or coach.

Jim Coleman—U.S.A. National Team Director
1968 U.S.A. Olympic Coach
1980 U.S.A. Men's Coach

Books in West's Physical Activities Series

Aerobics Today by Carole Casten and Peg Jordan
Aqua Aerobics Today by Carole Casten
Badminton Today by Tariq Wadood and Karlyne Tan
Dance Today by Lorraine Person, Judy Alter and Marian Weiser
Golf Today by J. C. Snead and John Johnson
Racquetball Today by Lynn Adams and Erwin Goldbloom
Swimming and Aquatics Today by Ron Ballatore and William Miller
Tennis Today by Glenn Bassett and William Otta
Volleyball Today by Marv Dunphy and Rod Wilde
Walk, Jog, Run Today by Jim Bush, Pat McArthur, and Eldin Onsgard
Weight Training Today by Robert O'Connor, Jerry Simmons and,
    J. Patrick O'Shea

The Series Editor for West's Physical Activities Series

The Series Editor for West's Physical Activities Series is Dr. Bob O'Connor, Los Angeles Pierce College. Dr. O'Connor received his B.S. and M.S. degrees in physical education from UCLA and his doctorate from USC. His 30-year teaching experience includes instruction in physical education courses of tennis, weight training, volleyball, badminton, swimming and various team sports, as well as classes in teaching methods. He brings to the Series a wide range of college coaching experience in areas of swimming, tennis, water polo, and football. Internationally, Dr. O'Connor has been an advisor to several Olympic programs in weight training and swimming. He was among the first to popularize strength training for all athletic events. Dr. O'Connor has written extensively in the fields of physical education and health and is a dedicated advocate of physical education TODAY.

CHAPTER 1

The Game of Volleyball

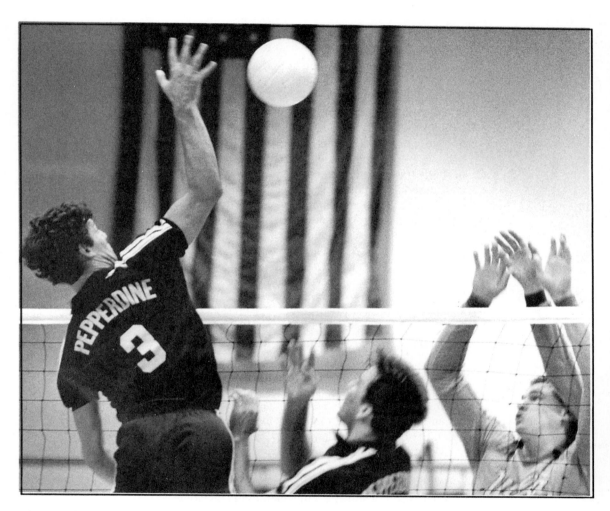

Outline

History
Popularity
Summary

Volleyball has become a very popular game in America and, indeed, throughout the world—it is second to only soccer in worldwide popularity. It is played from elementary school age through the senior citizen ranks. It is played with as few as two players per team to as many as six in official games, and sometimes even more in pickup games and at parties or picnics.

It is an international game that requires great skill and complex strategy, but it can be adapted to any level of play—and it is always fun.

History

The game was first developed by William G. Morgan, who had completed his degree in physical education at Springfield College (then known as the School for Christian Workers) in 1894. While working at a YMCA (Young Men's Christian Association) in Holyoke, Massachusetts, he attempted to get the local businessmen involved in the game of basketball, which had also been developed by a Springfield College man.

Morgan succeeded in getting some men to play basketball for recreation, but some of the older men did not like the game's roughness. Morgan then thought of just having them hit the basketball back and forth by hand. He also considered having them play tennis, but rejected that idea because the equipment required (balls, racquets, and nets) was too costly. But the concept of a net to divide the Players seemed like a good idea, so he put a net between two groups of participants. He decided to put the net at a height of six and one-half feet. (It is now near 8 feet.) Next he developed a few rules and a new game was created.

Games usually don't evolve in vacuums. The game of *minton* was probably familiar to Morgan—it might be considered a first cousin to volleyball. Minton was introduced in the United States in 1895. The game was played by two teams of four players who played on a 40 x 80 court and hit the ball over the net with a bat. The net was six and one-half feet high. The server would hit the ball over the net and a returner would have to immediately hit it back over. If the server's team failed to get the ball over, it was a fault and the server lost the serve. If the returners failed to return the ball, the serving team got a point. When all players on the serving team had lost their serves, the side would be out and the other team would get the serve. When both sides were out it was called the completion of an inning. Four innings constituted a game.[1]

Morgan's group first tried hitting a basketball, which was too heavy, and then a basketball bladder, which was too light and slow. Because the basketball was "too heavy and made our wrists sore, . . . we had Spaulding Company make us a ball made of soft calfskin which didn't last long."[2]

While Morgan said that he had no knowledge of any similar games, there were actually a few European sports that were somewhat like his. During the Middle Ages, groups of Italians played a game that had some similarities to volleyball. A modification of that game, introduced in Germany in 1893, was called *faust ball*.

---

[1]"Minton," *YMCA Athletic League Handbook* (New York: American Sports Publishing Company, 1897), p. 168.
[2]George O. Draper, "William C. Morgan—Inventor of Volleyball," *Official Volleyball Rules* (New York: American Sports Publishing Company, 1970), p. 41.

Morgan first called his game *mintonette*. The first exhibition of the game was at Springfield College on July 7, 1896. Among the participants at the first game were J. Curran and John Lynch, respectively the mayor and fire chief of Holyoke.

In 1896, Morgan was invited to give a demonstration of the game at a conference at Springfield College. He gave the presider a copy of the rules of the game—written in long hand.[3]

While watching the game at Springfield College, faculty member Alfred Halstead christened the game "volleyball." It seemed like a logical name because the ball was volleyed over the net.

The rules changed often. In the original game, as in today's game, the ball had to be volleyed, not caught, and the players could not touch the net. Any number of people could play, and players could reach over or go under the net. The court size was not standardized, and players did not rotate.

In 1896, W. E. Day introduced the new sport at Dayton, Ohio. He developed some new rules. Among the rule changes were that the net was raised to seven and one-half feet, eliminating the possibility of dribbling the ball (multiple hits by one player), and that the game was standardized at 21 points.

The more modern version of the rules started in 1912. The court size and the ball were standardized, and the rule requiring the players to rotate before a serve was instituted. In 1916, the YMCA and the NCAA (National Collegiate Athletic Association) published the rules of the game and made additional changes. They set the height of the net at eight feet, set the game score at 15, and made the winner of the match the team that won two out of three games.

In the early 1920s, A. Provost Idell and his teammates added a few more rules. They standardized the court at 30 x 60 feet, established the rule limiting the number of hits per side to three, and required that the ball be played only from above the waist.

Popularity

The game began to become popular. The game was introduced to the Philippines in 1910, to Japan in 1913, to Poland in 1915, to Uruguay in 1916, to Brazil and Latvia in 1919, and to Syria in 1922. After World War I, it was introduced throughout Europe.

While the YMCA kept volleyball as an indoor game, the Playground of America (now the National Recreation Association) started to teach it as an outdoor game after the Playground of America's 1907 convention.

In the early 1920s, the University of Illinois began to teach volleyball as a physical education activity. The university also began an intramural program featuring volleyball competition.

The first college team was formed by the University of Oregon in 1928. The University of Washington followed with a team in 1934. These teams played in recreational leagues. The first university volleyball league began in 1941 with 12 teams, among them teams from Columbia, Temple, and the University of Pennsylvania.

---

[3]Ibid.

By the late 1940s many colleges fielded club teams, and by 1952 the NCAA was willing to sponsor national championships if eight schools were ready to field varsity teams. While many colleges fielded club teams, only six were ready with varsity teams at that time.

The United States Volleyball Association (USVBA) was formed in 1928, and by 1937 it controlled the game in the United States. In 1947, the International Volleyball Federation was formed to regulate the game throughout the world. Fifteen nations sent representatives. (Today there are over 150 members.) In 1953 the first World Championships were held, in 1955 volleyball was played in the first Pan American Games, and in 1964 it became an Olympic sport.

The popularity of the game today is evidenced by the rapid increase in players. A recent Gallup poll showed that 34 million Americans had played volleyball at least once in the last year. Of the 50 sports listed in the survey, volleyball was the twelfth most popular sport. Further, the polled showed that in the last 25 years the sport had increased in popularity by 500 percent and that it is growing even more rapidly today. In fact, more people participate in volleyball than in tennis, soccer, skiing, racquetball, golf, or baseball.

While the game is most popular among the 25 to 35 age group, it is quickly attracting a following among the young. During the last five years youth volleyball has doubled in popularity and is the fastest-growing sport among young Americans. Interscholastic volleyball is the third most popular sport for girls; and boys' teams are rapidly being implemented across the country. In one recent year over 50 boys' teams were instituted in New York City alone!

As spectator sports, the international game and the beach game continue to attract fans both at the game and via television. And as the spectators' knowledge of the game increases, the demand increases for more games.

Summary

1. The game of volleyball was invented by William Morgan, a graduate of Springfield College—the same college at which basketball was invented.
2. The game began as a non-contact recreational pastime.
3. The modern rules were fairly well established by the early 1920s.
4. Volleyball is a sport whose popularity is rapidly growing both as a participant sport and as a spectator sport.

CHAPTER 2

Facilities and Equipment

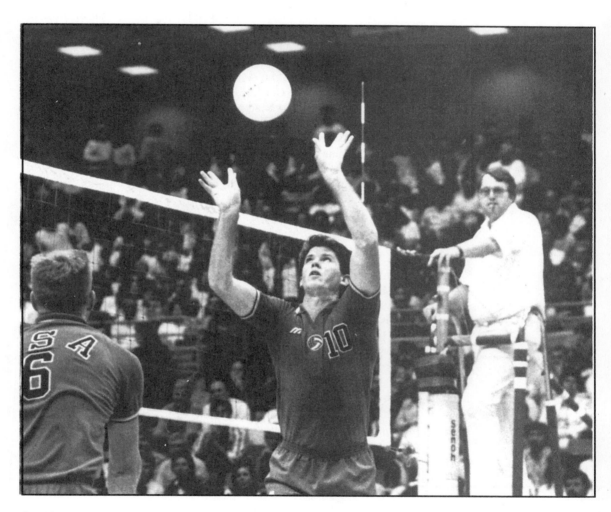

Outline

The Court

The traditional American court is 30 x 60 feet, with a ceiling height of at least 23 feet. With the exception of international matches, most games in the United States are played on this traditional court.

The international court is 59 feet (18 meters) long and 29½ feet wide (nine meters). It is bounded by lines two inches wide. The outside edge of the lines marks the outside perimeter of the court, so the lines are considered inside the court and balls that hit the lines are considered "in." This is different from some games, such as football, where the lines are considered "out."

There is another line—the center line—which bisects the court into two sections. The net goes over this line. Also, there is a line on each side of the court running parallel to the net (and center line), three meters from the center line. This is called the "three meter line," the "back court spiking line," or the "attack line." The three players whose positions were in the back court at the serve cannot send the ball over the net, if they are above the height of the net. The exception being when their jump was initiated from beyond the three meter line. This restrains a team from having its best spiker always playing in the front line.

The serving area is behind the end line and within three meters (ten feet) of the right sideline (as the server faces the net).

The Net

The net is slightly longer than the width of the court; 32 feet is common length. Most nets are 36 inches from top to bottom, with the cords (made of nylon or other fibers) spaced three to four inches apart so that there is a rather wide-mesh (as opposed to a tennis net, which has a narrow mesh). There is a wire nylon cable of ⅛- to ⅜-inch diameter that runs through the top binding of the net. This allows the net to be pulled tightly, so that it is nearly straight across.

When set up, the middle of the net will be 7 feet, 11⅝ inches (2.43 meters) high for men. For women, the net height is 7 feet, 4¼ inches or 7 feet, 4⅛ inches (2.24 meters).

The bottom binding of the net will also be securely anchored. This allows balls that are hit into the net to bounce outward and remain in play.

The Standards

The standards that support the net are mounted in the floor in some gyms. This is the best and safest type of standard. Many gyms have standards that rest on a base on the floor. These require additional anchoring with guy wires set into the floor or the walls.

The Referee's Stand

The referee's stand is generally attached to one of the standards and allows the referee to stand about four feet above floor level. From this vantage point the official can better see the play at the net and can call net touching and illegal movements over or under the net.

The Antennae

In official games a thin pole, usually fiberglass, is extended over each sideline from the top of the net to a level three feet above the net. The antennae are there to assist the officials and players in determining whether or not the ball passed over the net in bounds (inside the antenna). If a team does not hit the ball over the net in bounds, the ball is not in play.

The Ball

The official ball is made of leather and is 25 to 27 inches in circumference. The ball is generally white, but can be off-white or even yellow—a color often used for beach volleyball. Indoor volleyball is played with a white ball. Because of the cost of leather and the fact that school volleyball is often played outside, manufacturers have developed both synthetic leather balls and rubber balls. The synthetic leather balls cost about half of what the leather balls cost, and the rubber balls cost only about a quarter as much as leather balls. The rubber balls also wear better than the leather balls when the game is played on asphalt or concrete.

Clothing

Shorts and Shirt

A player's shorts and shirt should fit loosely, to allow a full range of movement. They should also allow for absorption of perspiration—a blend of 50 percent cotton and 50 percent polyester makes an effective fabric.

Socks

Cotton gym socks should be sufficient. Two pairs of socks will help to reduce the possibility of getting blisters, because the socks will rub against each other and absorb the friction that might otherwise be transferred to your skin.

Shoes

At the lower levels of play, nearly any court shoe should be sufficient. The shoes should be pliable, well cushioned, and have good traction. A heel and toe lock will lengthen the life of the shoe. The shoe should also be somewhat rounded to allow for lateral movements. If you are playing indoors, the shoes should have soles that will not mark the floor. At the higher levels of play, you may want to buy shoes specifically designed for volleyball.

Checklist For Footgear

1. Whether wearing one or two pairs of socks, pull them up tight so that no wrinkles will remain (these might cause blisters).
2. When lacing the shoes, pull the laces tight at the lowest eyelets. Then slowly pull the laces tight at each eyelet upward until the laces have been adjusted at each level. Then they should be tied.
3. Just slipping on your shoes and pulling the laces from the top does not adjust the shoes properly for an action game such as volleyball. Improper lacing can create blisters.

Sweat Clothes

When warming up or when playing on cold days, sweat clothing should be worn. The muscles react better and are less susceptible to injury when they are kept warm. Consequently, sweats can be worn during game warmups and should be worn between games or when one is waiting to play. A hooded sweatshirt without a zipper is considered best for volleyball.

Pads

For players who dive for balls, both knee and elbow pads may be worn. They reduce the chance of developing bone bruises or abrasions from contact with the floor. Hip pads are another type of optional equipment that help reduce the chance of injury.

Sweatbands

Some players use sweatbands to keep the perspiration from dropping into their eyes. Sweatbands may also be used to keep the hair away from one's face.

Other Considerations

Jewelry shouldn't be worn during play (the official rules forbid it)—for example, a bracelet or wristwatch may break if hit with the ball. Hard objects, such as casts, should also not be worn.

Summary

1. The international court is 18 x 9 meters. The lines are in bounds.
2. The net height is 7 feet, 11$5/8$ inches in the center of the net for men's volleyball and 7 feet, 4$1/8$ inches for the women's game.
3. Players should wear comfortable clothing (shorts and shirts), perspiration-absorbent socks, and court shoes with good traction and effective shock-absorbing ability.
4. For their safety players may wear knee, elbow, and hip pads to prevent injuries, and sweat clothes to prevent pulled muscles.

CHAPTER 3

Rules, Regulations, and Terminology

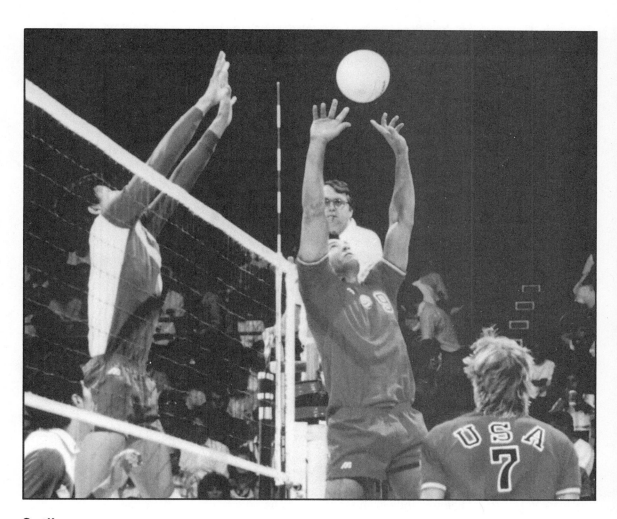

Outline

Rules
Terminology
Summary
Checklist for Overlap

Rules often change, so players must keep current. For example, it was once allowed to kick the ball; that is no longer legal. It was once required that players stay in prescribed areas during a serve; now it is required only that they not overlap each other. At one time players were not allowed to cross the plane of the net; now, with certain limitations, they can go over or under as long as they do not touch the net.

The rules vary somewhat from international and college rules to high school, coed, or beach rules. The following rules are for the international and college levels of play. However, there are other sanctioning bodies that also make rules. The NAGWS (National Association for Girls' and Women's Sports) formulates the rules for most collegiate women's programs and for some high school girls' competition.

Rules

A *team* is made up of six players. Generally, a squad will have a total of 12 players on the roster; however, some leagues and conferences allow for a variation in this roster rule.

An *official game* is concluded when one team has scored 15 points and has won by two points. In USVBA, international, and in men's intercollegiate rules, the game is "capped" when a team reaches 17 points, even if it is only one point ahead. Other levels of play have not yet adopted this rule.

The deciding game in a five-game match is a fast-scoring (rally point scoring) game. This means that both teams can score at any time. The serving team scores as it always does, but the receiving team also gains a point when it gets a side out. This obviously speeds up the deciding game.

A *match* is won when one team has won three games out of five or, in a "short match," when one team has won two games out of three.

Flipping the coin for choice of side or serve is done by the captains before the first game and again before the fifth game if a fifth game is needed. (For games two through four, *opening service* is alternated—the team receiving opening serve in game one delivers opening serve in game two, and so on.) The winning captain can choose to serve or to start the game on a preferred side of the court. The position of the sun or a glare from windows might prompt a captain to choose "side" rather than "serve."

Points are scored only by the serving team. They are scored when the opponents have committed a violation or fail to win the rally. (As previously stated, in "fast-scoring" either team can score on any serve.)

Side out occurs when the serving team commits a foul or hits the ball out of bounds, thus losing its serve. The opposing team then becomes the serving team.

Positions and zones are named to identify where players are to be during a serve or to determine where a set will be directed or a spike will be hit. The players in the three front zones are called the *right front* (zone 2), *center front* (zone 3), and *left front* (zone 4). The three back row players are the *left back* (zone 5), the *center back* (zone 6), and the server (if the team has the serve) or *right back* (if the team is receiving) (zone 1).

Rotations occur just after a side out as the new server moves from the right front (zone 2) to the right back (zone 1). Players rotate clockwise.

Two *time outs* are allowed to each team per game. Time outs are 30 seconds long.

Substitutions may enter the game only one time under USVBA rules. The player who was replaced by the substitute must take his or her original position if he or she returns to the game. A starting player can be replaced only one time per game. The substitute cannot return to the game once he or she has been replaced by the original player. There is a six substitution limit under the USVBA rules. Most other levels of volleyball allow for 12 substitutions per game.

A *contact* occurs any time the ball hits the body at a point above and including the waist. (A contact below the waist would be a violation.) The ball can be contacted three times on each side of the net; a fourth contact would be a violation. So a pass, a set, and then an attack would be the three normal contacts a team would make. Note that the ball can also be legally hit over the net with fewer than three contacts. A ball touched by the block is not counted as one of the three contacts.

Fouls or violations result in a side out if committed by the serving team. If they are committed by the receiving team, they result in a point for the serving team.

A violation of any of the following at time of serve results in a sideout:

- When the serve is gained, the serving team players rotate clockwise, and the player entering the right back position is the new server.
- The serve must be hit by the right back court player.
- It must be hit from an area behind the end line and the server must not be farther than three meters (ten feet) to the left of the extension of the side-line. A mark on the end line denotes this service area.
- The server may not step on the back line until after the ball has been contacted.
- The ball must be tossed into the air prior to contacting it with the serving hand.
- The ball must be hit with the hand (although it may be in any manner).
- The serve cannot hit the net.
- The serve must pass over the net between the antennae.
- Only one service attempt is allowed. (However, if the server drops the ball without hitting it, it is not considered a violation, and he or she is allowed one more opportunity.)
- The serve must land on or between the lines of the receiver's court or be contacted by a player on the receiving team in order to be a legal serve.
- During a serve or service return, a player may not overlap an adjacent player. Thus a back row player cannot be as near the net as the front row player in the zone ahead. Also, a player cannot overlap the player in the zone to the side. Once the serve is contacted the players may move any-where, but back row players cannot block or spike from ahead of the three meter line.
- A served ball cannot be blocked or spiked by the receiving team. The serving team is awarded a point if this occurs.

A violation of any of the following with the ball in play results in a side out if committed by the serving team or in a point if committed by the receiving team:

- Each contact must give the ball immediate impetus—the ball must be clearly hit, not lifted, scooped, or thrown.
- A player may not hit the ball twice in succession (a double hit), unless it is the first contact or the first contact was a block or a simultaneous hit with another player.
- The ball may be played with any part of the body above the waist, but cannot contact any part of the body below the waist.
- If opponents hit the ball simultaneously, either one can hit it again.
- If teammates hit the ball simultaneously, neither can play the next contact.
- The ball may not be hit more than three times in succession by the players of one team, unless the first contact was a block (which does not count as one of the three allowed contacts).
- If any part of the ball is over the net it can be contacted by either team.
- The ball must land within the opponents' court or touch any part of the boundary line in order to be called in bounds.
- Players may not touch the net unless it has been driven into them; the ball, however, may touch the net and remain in play (except for a served ball).
- Players may shift positions after the ball has been served, but a player who was in the back row at the time of the service cannot spike or block the ball from inside of the three meter line.
- A ball coming over the net, may not be spiked unless part of it has crossed the net. It cannot be touched if it is still on the opponent's side of the net unless the opponent has made the third contact or the ball is clearly going to pass over the net (then it can be blocked).
- Blockers may reach over the net to block a spike after it has been hit. They cannot block a set.
- A player may not play the ball outside the court if it has completely crossed the center line extended. A player can play under the net if the ball has been hit there by one of his or her teammates and has not completely crossed the center line.
- The ball may be played by a player who is out of bounds, but it must cross the net in bounds (completely inside the antennae or the vertical extension of the antennae) in order to be legal.
- No part of the body, other than the foot, may touch the opponent's court. The foot may touch the opponent's court but some part of the foot must be in contact with the center line.

A point must be *replayed* in either of the following instances:

- If two opponents simultaneously hit a ball and the ball is stopped or held.
- If the two teams make simultaneous fouls.

Terminology

Arc—Trajectory of the ball. A pass to a setter who is close would have a sharper, more pronounced arc than would a ball passed to a player who is more distant.

Attack—Hitting the ball into the opponent's court. The most common attacking hit is the *spike*.

Attack line—The line on the court that is 9 feet, 10 inches (three meters) from the center line.

Attacker—The person who hits the ball over the net.

Back set—A set that goes to a spot behind the setter.

Block—An attempt by one to three front row players to stop an attacked ball. The blockers jump and extend their arms over the net, attempting to block the ball down onto the opponents court.

Bump—An underhanded, two-armed pass in which the ball rebounds from the forearms and is directed to a teammate.

Center line—The line directly under the net that separates the two halves of the court.

Contacts or ball contacts—Are counted every time a player touches the ball. Three contacts are permitted, but no player can hit the ball twice in succession. The exception to this rule is when a player has blocked a ball at the net: When this occurs, the team will still be allowed three more contacts and the blocking player can hit the ball on the first contact, immediately after the block. If a ball hits a player, even if unintentionally, it is a contact and counts as one of the three allowed ball contacts. If two players hit a ball simultaneously, it is considered one contact.

Cross-court spike—A spike directed across the court to the greatest diagonal distance.

Dig—A one- or two-handed pass made from an opponent's attack.

Dink—A soft shot made by the spiker who with open hand, guides the ball just over the arms of the blockers. It can be done with one or two hands and is made from the fingertips. Also called a *tip*.

Double fault—A violation committed by players on both teams simultaneously. The point is replayed.

Down-the-line spike—A spike made close to the near sideline, rather than diagonally.

Floater—A serve hit without spin that may move up, down, or sideways depending on how the air pressure builds in front of the ball.

Forearm pass—Same as a *bump*; the most-used skill in volleyball.

Free ball—A ball hit over the net that is not spiked.

Heel of the hand—The fleshy part of the hand just above the wrist.

Lateral pass—A pass played from the side of the body when time does not allow the passer to play the ball from the body's midline.

Line of flight—The ball's direction after a pass or set.

Middle back-up—A defensive alignment in which one player plays behind the block to protect against a dinked ball.

Netting—Touching the net while the ball is in play.

Off hand—A spike in which the ball must be hit with the hand away from the place where it was set. For example, for a ball to be hit from the left side of a right-handed spiker, it must cross the body and then be hit.

On hand—A ball set from the same side as the spiker's favored hand.

Opening up—Occurs on a served ball when the players recognize which teammate will receive it and face (open up to) the passer to enable him or her to take the pass.

Overhand pass—A pass played with open hands to put the ball up to the net for a set.

Pass—The first contact after the ball has come over the net.

Penetrate—Moving the arms across the net when blocking—the airspace of the opponents is being penetrated.

Power alley—The area most likely to receive a spike; usually the diagonal area from where the spike is hit, inside the block.

Quick hit—A spike made from a low set with the objective of beating a block before it is formed or fooling a blocker because of the quickness.

Rally—Occurs when the teams are hitting the ball back and forth across the net more than one time.

Reverse set—same as *back set*.

Rotation—Occurs before every serve when each member of the new serving team moves one position clockwise—the front line moves one position to the right, the right front player moves to the right back and becomes the server, the back-row players move one position left, and the left back-row player moves forward to become the leftmost player in the front line.

Seal—Occurs when there is no space between the blocker's arms and the top of the net.

Seam—The area between two receivers on a serve, or the area between two blockers.

Serve—The act of putting the ball in play by hitting it with one hand from behind the end line in the serving area.

Serving area—The ten-foot area from the right sideline inward, from which the serve must be hit.

Set—Generally the second contact on a side. The ball is contacted with all the pads of the fingers of both hands simultaneously. The ball may have a momentary rest on the fingers, but if it is held it is considered a violation. The set should be placed exactly to the point most advantageous to the spiker.

Setter(s)—The one or more designated players who are responsible for making the set to the attacker.

Shaping the hands—Refers to the hand position when setting.

Side out—Occurs when the serving team for whatever reason does not score a point, and thus service goes to the opponent.

Spike—Generally hit after the ball is set. It must be hit from spiker's side of the net, but the spiker's hand and arm may follow through across the net.

Sprawl—A technique used to get to a low serve or spike.

Target area—The area toward which the pass is directed. The setter is released into this area to prepare to set.

Tip—Same as dink.

Transition—The term for changing from offense to defense or defense to offense.

Underhand pass—Same as a *bump*.

Volley—An overhand pass or set.

Wipeoff—An offensive shot that is brushed off the blocker's arms and then goes out of bounds.

Zones—Some teams use a numbering system to indicate the placement of a player or the target area of the ball. A common numbering system designates the back right third of the court (the area of the server) as zone 1. Zone 2 is the right front court. Zone 3 is the middle front third of the court. Zone 4 is the left front third. Zone 5 is the left back area, and zone 6 is the middle back area.

Summary

1. There are six players on a regulation volleyball team.
2. A game ends at 15 points, but must be won by two points. Thus it would be possible to have a game ending at 21–19, or even 30–28. Men's Collegiate and USVBA rules now have a 17-point cap on the game, so a game could be won 17–16.
3. A team can score points only when it is serving, unless the match encompasses fast scoring for the fifth game.
4. When a serving team commits a violation it is a side out and the other team gains the serve.
5. Three contacts (not counting a contact by a blocker) are allowed before the ball must cross the net.
6. The ball can be played with any part of the body above the waist.
7. The rules often change so the player must keep current on the rule updates.

Checklist for Overlap

1. During a serve, before the ball is contacted, the players may not overlap an adjacent player.
   a. The left front player must be positioned so that the left back player is behind and the center front player is to the right.
   b. The center front player must be ahead of the center back player and must not overlap the left or the right front players.
   c. The right front player must be ahead of the right back player and not overlap the center front player.
   d. The left back player must not be ahead of the left front player and must not overlap the center back player.
   e. The center back player must not line up ahead of the center front player nor overlap either of the other back row players.
   f. The right back player (server) must not be positioned ahead of the right front player nor overlap the center back player.
2. Once the serve is contacted, the players may move to any desired position as long as a back row player does not attempt to block or attack from in front of the three meter line.

Forearm Passing or Bumping

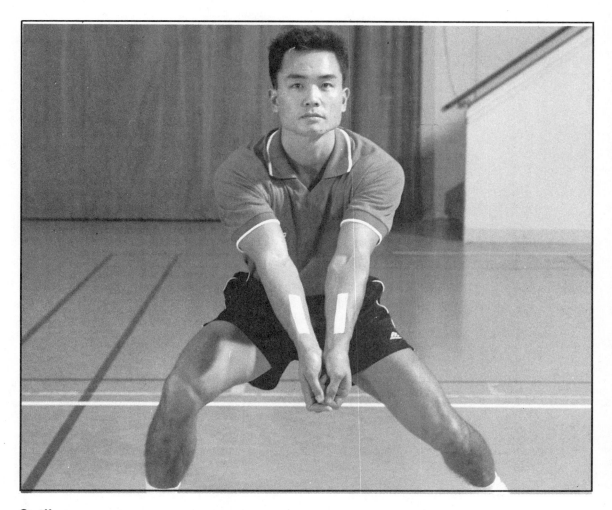

Outline

Passing is the term used to denote the first regular contact of a team after the ball has crossed the net on a serve or other type of hit. The pass is directed to the setter. The setter will then set to the attacker.

The forearm pass is the most frequently used skill in the game of volleyball. It is, therefore, a very important skill and should be learned first. Without some mastery of this skill, volleyball cannot be played well at any level. The forearm pass is used to receive service, to dig spikes, and in other situations when the player cannot get in a good position to pass the ball overhand.

The forearm pass, or *bump*, should be hit high enough and accurately enough to allow the setter time to make a good set to the attacker.

Making the Pass

When possible, the player should move his or her body in line with the flight of the ball so that the ball can be played forward of the body and at the body's midline. Slide to a position in front of the ball. Do not cross your legs when moving sideways, unless there is a long distance to be covered. Also remember to keep your feet on the ground. Never lift your feet to make a pass—the legs act as shock absorbers, not propellants.

Try to keep your body movement to a minimum, since there is really very little time to move if the serve is hard or you are playing a spiked ball. Players in women's leagues may need a lower stance than those in men's leagues, as the ball may come in at a sharper angle because of the lower net.

The passer should play the ball low. The knees should be flexed with the feet apart slightly wider than shoulder width. The feet should be staggered with the right foot forward. It is possible when passing at an angle for the foot closest to the direction of the pass to be slightly forward. For example, if the passer is on the outside edge of the court and is directing the pass forward and toward the center, the outside foot can be set back to make it easier for the passer to aim the pass back into the court by shifting his or her weight or striding toward the target area.

Starting position

Side view of receiving posture

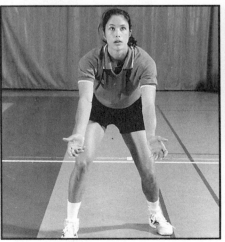
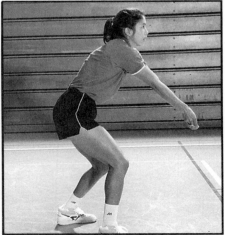

a.

b.

c.

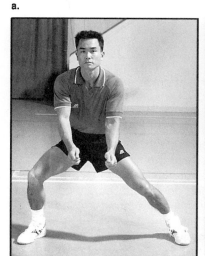
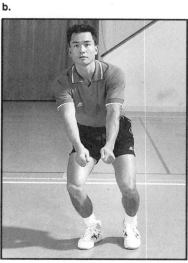
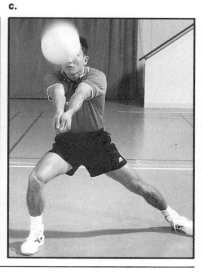

a. passer moving
laterally to ball,
b. passer not
crossing legs during
movement,
c. re-establishing
wide base with right
foot forward

The back should be bent slightly forward and the head should be slightly down. With the head down, the eyes can follow the ball almost to the point of contact on the forearms. With the weight carried forward the passer should feel more weight on the toes, particularly on the inside toes.

To make the *passing platform* the arms should be straight, elbows locked, and the heels of the hands (near the wrist) touching each other. Both hands will be pointing toward the floor, so that the fleshy part of the forearms is exposed. The radius bone (the long bone from the elbow to the thumb side of the wrist) is rotated outward, so that the ball will not contact it. This gives a wider platform area with which to control the ball. The ball should be contacted two to six inches above the wrists.

a. close up forearm
platform with contact
points, b. ball on
contact points

a.

b.

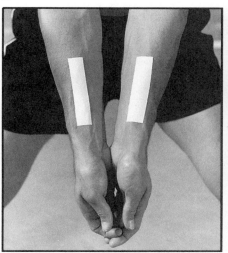
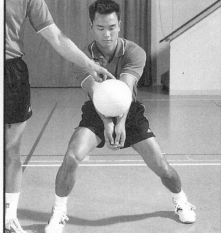

Checklist for the Pass

1. The feet will be set apart wider than the shoulders, with the right foot forward.
2. The back should be bent forward and the head should be down with the eyes focused on the ball.
3. The knees should be bent to whatever angle is necessary to be able to play the ball between the waist and the knees.
4. With the elbows locked and the hands interlocking and with the heels of the hands touching and pointed downward, gently guide the ball toward the target area. The angle of the arms to the floor will determine the arc of the ball.
5. Set the angle of the platform prior to contacting the ball.
6. The body weight should shift forward toward the target as the ball is contacted. This assists in achieving the proper trajectory.

The key to making a flat platform with the forearms is to have the bases of the hands touching and even—neither higher than the other. The fingers are usually overlapped in this position, but they may be slightly interlocked or even separated from each other as long as the arms do not break apart. Note that the fingers should not form a fist.

Rather than swinging at the ball, the arms should be used as a platform so that the ball will rebound in the proper direction and with the desired arc. It is important to "set the angle" of the platform prior to contacting the ball. Think soft—softly shovel and guide the ball into your target area. The harder the spike or serve is hit at you, the more you must absorb the speed of the ball while making the pass.

The body and arms will move slightly forward as the pass, or bump, is made. The ball should be contacted at a height between the waist and the knees.

Front view of passing posture with contact points visible

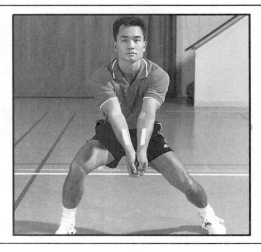

Side view of passing posture with contact

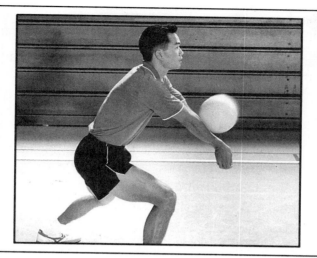

The angle of the arms from the shoulder will determine the arc of the ball. It is a law of physics that the angle of incidence equals the angle of refraction. So if a ball is coming at a 30° angle to the lower part of the arm, it will leave at a 30° angle to the upper part of the arm. With practice you will begin to feel the proper angle of the arms for the desired arc of the pass. Generally, an angle of approximately 45° to the floor will be best.

As the pass is made, shift your weight in the direction of the target. A shuffle step with the lead foot can also assist the ball in the direction of the target.

The *height* of the pass is the most difficult thing to control. A pass that is too high may cause problems for the attacker and thus give the defense time to get set. Generally, a pass should follow an arc high enough to allow the setter to get into position and to set the ball. The target area should be about two and one-half feet from the net.

Anticipate your play by being aware of your position on the court and where your target area will be. Then concentrate on the opponent's server—always expect the ball to come to you. Be "fast to the ball" once you have determined the direction of the serve or spike. It is important to get behind the ball quickly rather than under the ball quickly.

Analyze the server's style. Does the server use a top spin serve or a jump serve that will dive quickly after it crosses the net? If so, position yourself closer to the net to be able to play the dropping ball. Does the server like to serve down the line or crosscourt? Position yourself to best be able to handle the expected serve.

Concentration is a major factor. Your eyes must be on the person hitting the ball—the server or spiker. The point of contact and the follow through will give you an idea as to the direction and the speed of the ball. Since it takes about a half a second for an elite volleyball player to see the ball and react with the arms, you can understand why it is so important to concentrate on the hitter instead of the ball and save perhaps a fraction of a second in reaction time. Most beginners wait until they see the ball in flight before they begin to make their preparations for the pass.

Checklist for Common Errors in Passing

1. Establishing the forearm platform too late.
2. Making the platform too close to the body.
3. Bending or swinging the platform.
4. Contacting the ball too low on the forearms or wrists.

Types of Passes

The *pass off the serve* is difficult because the serve is generally coming hard and may be coming with a spin, or, in the case of a float serve, it may move in an unpredictable way. The one advantage for the receiver is that he or she has more time to prepare for this pass than when playing a spiked ball.

Extended stride to receive short ball

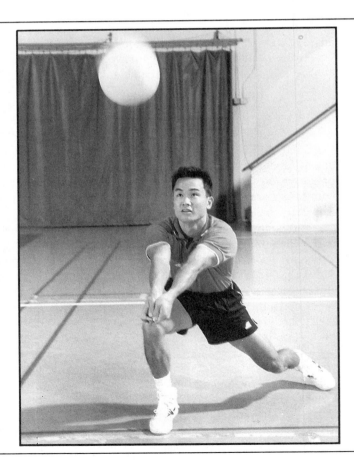

Preparing for lateral pass

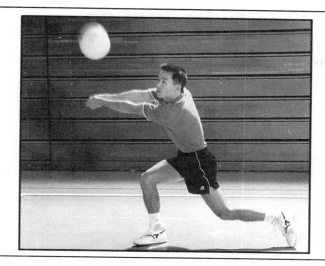

A *pass to a moving setter* who is switching positions occurs at every level of play. The pass must be made to the target area into which the setter will move slightly in front of the setter.

A *pass directly to a front court setter/attacker* is occasionally done at the elite level of play to reduce the effectiveness of a block. The passer passes directly to the setter/attacker, who may then spike the ball.

A *lateral pass* is sometimes required. Because of the spontaneous nature of the game, it is not always possible to make a perfect pass from the midline of the body. When the ball is to the side of the passer and the passer is unable to pass the ball from the body's midline, a lateral pass must be attempted. The player should step to a position with a trailing foot, thus allowing a weight shift to occur. The ball should still be played before it crosses the plane of the body.

Executing lateral pass

Passing a high ball

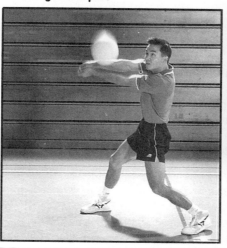

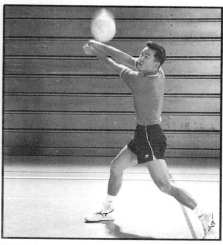

Because the ball is being played outside of the midline of the body, it must be played farther in front of the body to ensure the proper angle required to complete the pass.

In the lateral pass the forearm platform is maintained as in a regular pass, but the arms are extended to the side of the body. The platform will be angled so that the ball can be directed from the contact point at the side of the body toward the target area. This is done by lifting the arm farthest from the target and tilting the platform forward toward the target.

The *highball pass* is necessary when the ball cannot be played low. It can be done with open hands, as in a set (see Chapter 5), or with a reverse forearm pass. However, it is difficult to play a hard-hit ball with open hands and not be called for a double contact or for holding it.

The reverse forearm pass is executed when the ball is at chest height or higher. The passer flexes the knees if necessary so that the pass can be taken at head height. The hands and forearms are kept in the same relative position as in a low pass, but the elbows are at about head height and pointed forward. The ball is contacted on the back of the forearms on the ulnar bone (the bone that is on the same side of the arm as the little finger) and angled upward and toward the target area.

Practice for passing is best done by receiving serves. While beginning drills will be performed with one person tossing the ball softly to the passer, realistic game drills will be practiced by returning serves.

When *receiving the serve* it must be remembered that while the ball will travel slower than a spiked ball, it will often change directions because of the buildup of air pressure in front of the ball. It may move up, down, or to the side. In fact, it may make several such movements during the flight from the server.

Watch the server to determine the angle of the follow through and the action of the wrist to be able to get the jump on the ball.

Front-row players should not play balls that are above waist level. Leave them for the back-court players. If the ball is played by a front-row player, the back-row players must back up the play in case the ball is not passed perfectly. Back-row players should play 60 percent to 70 percent of the balls.

Drills

1. Any drill that has the ball coming over the net.
2. Triangle passing drill has a server, passer and a target. The target person catches the passed ball and throws it to the server.
3. (Pairs) Partners pass to each other.
4. (Pairs) Each partner gets two hits in a row—a bump to oneself, then a bump back to the partner. Variations include:

   a. Bump to self, then bump to partner.
   b. Bump to self, make a quarter turn, then bump to partner.
   c. Bump to self, make a half turn, then bump to partner.
   d. Bump to self, make a full turn, then bump to partner.

Triangle passing
The three players
forming the triangle
can rotate on time
or criteria established
by the instructor.

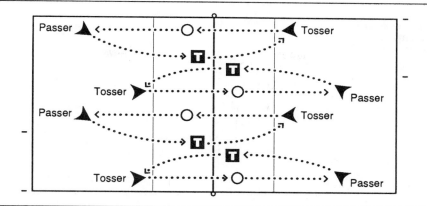

Partner passing

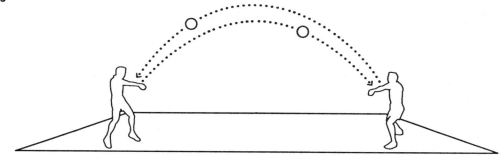

**Pass to self-pass to
partner**

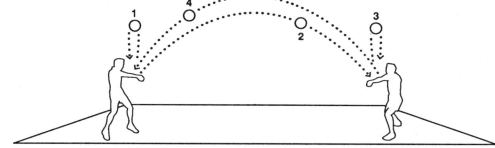

**Pass to self-1/4
turn-pass to
partner**

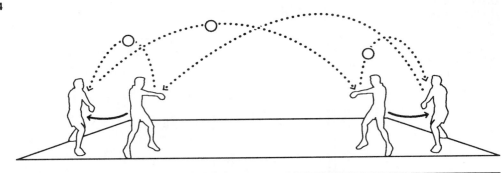

**Pass to self-1/2
turn-pass to
partner**

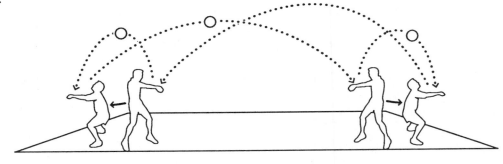

**Pass to self-full
turn-pass to
partner**

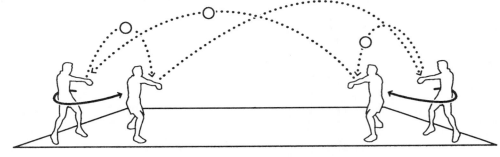

**Pass-squat-pass-
pass to partner**

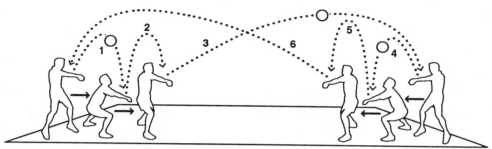

Pass-Pass-Pass

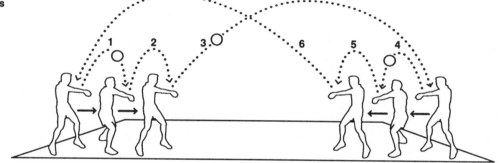

Team-serve-receive
Players can rotate
on time or criteria
designed by the
instructor. The
instructor should
insure some degree
of success.

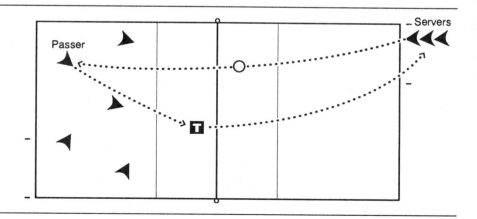

5. (Pairs) Each partner gets three hits in succession. Variations include:

    a. Bump to self, squat and make an overhand pass (set) to self, then bump to partner.
    b. Bump to self, squat and bump to self, bump to partner.
    c. (Intermediate and advanced players) Bump to self, do a forward roll, bump to self again, then bump to partner.

6. (Pairs) Partner alternates throwing the ball to the passer—at different heights, different directions (right and left), and different speeds—throwing harder as the player becomes more adept at passing.

7. (Pairs or teams) One side serves while the receivers make passes to a target or to a setter.

8. Pass a ball coming from the other side of the net, first thrown, then served, then spiked.

 Checklist for Learning Progression

Beginner skills:
1. Toss to the passer.
2. Pass to a stationary target/setter.
3. Pass from a serve.

Intermediate skills:
4. Lateral pass (outside midline of body).
5. High ball pass (above midline of body).
6. Pass to a moving setter.

Advanced skills:
7. Low trajectory pass.
8. Pass to setter/attacker.

Summary

1. Passing the ball is the primary skill necessary for success in volleyball.
2. The pass is used to get the ball in play after the opponents have served or have returned the ball.
3. The pass is made with the arms extended.
4. The passer must concentrate on the ball from the time it leaves the hands of the server or attacker.

CHAPTER 5

Setting and the Overhand Pass

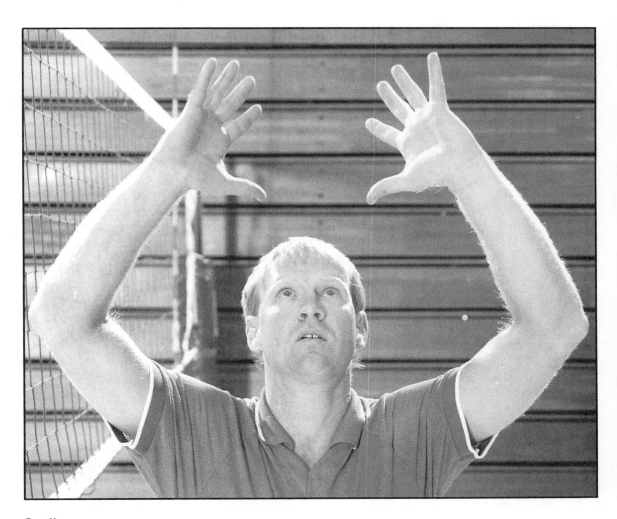

Outline

The set is generally an overhand pass that is directed to the point where the attacker can best hit it for a kill. The setter is expected to make a perfect set to the attacker so that the attacker can make the most effective play possible. Because passers often make poor passes, the setter should be a gifted athlete who is capable of running down errant passes.

The overhand pass should be used whenever possible (except on serve reception and when digging), because it is a very accurate method of passing the ball. It can be legally used on any shot, but it is very difficult to execute without making a double contact if the ball is coming fast, as in a serve or spike.

Techniques of the Overhand Pass

Get behind the ball as quickly as possible. Watch the passer in order to get an early tip on the direction and height of the pass. If you can't be standing in one spot when the pass arrives at least try to stop your body by shuffling to the spot, and stop momentarily even though your momentum is moving you. It is best not to set while running.

Drawing the hands to the setting position is done by bringing the hands quickly upward along the front of the body to a position directly above the upturned forehead. Beginners often bring their hands away from the body. This causes the setter to make contact with the ball in different areas above the forehead.

The hands are *shaped* by spreading the fingers and cupping them. They should be formed so that they will cup the ball when it contacts them. When ready to contact the ball, the index fingers and thumbs should form a triangle. The tips of the thumbs should be one to three inches apart and the tips of the index fingers should be two to four inches apart. (This varies with the size of the hands—players with smaller hands should hold them farther apart.) The thumbs should point slightly back toward the forehead.

**Overhand pass:
a. in position to set,
b. drawing up of the hands, c. hands drawn and shaped,
d. side view of hands drawn and shaped**

a.   b.   c.   d.

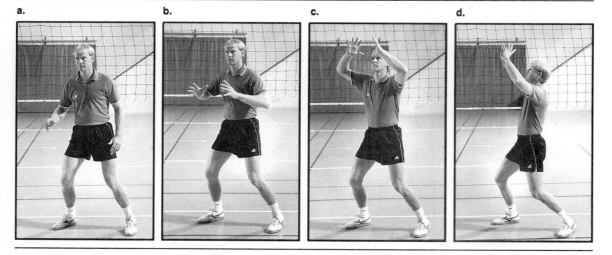

**Front and back views
of hands forming
triangle**

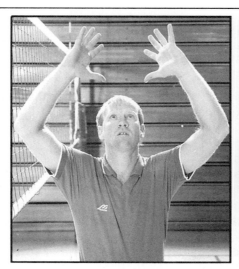
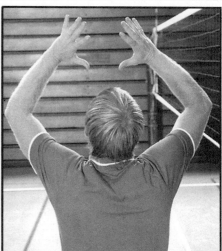

    The actual point of contact will be the pads of the fingers and thumbs—about an inch back from the fingertips. All of the fingers should touch the ball, but most of the pressure will be felt on the thumbs and forefingers. The outside fingers will help to control the ball.

    The fingers should be somewhat rigid, yet flexible. They should not be so stiff that the ball rebounds immediately nor so relaxed that the ball settles into the hands and is illegally caught.

    The *wrists* and *forearms* act as shock absorbers, because they absorb the weight and force of the ball and then launch it again into flight. The wrists should be in a comfortable, hyperextended (bent toward the back of the forearms) position as the ball approaches. The arms, not the wrists, supply the power. Because of this, forearm strength is necessary for good setting.

**Front and back views
of triangle with ball**

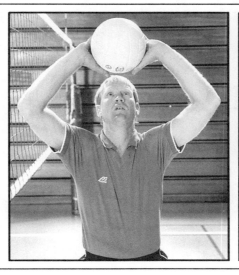
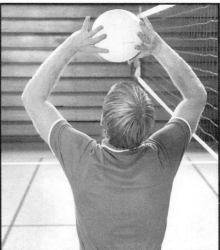

Checklist for the Overhand Set

1. The feet should be slightly staggered about shoulder-width apart, with the right foot forward.
2. The body should be bent slightly forward.
3. The upper arms should be parallel with the floor.
4. The hands should be in front of and above the upturned forehead.
5. The hands should be shaped for the ball and the wrists turned back so that the thumbs point toward the forehead.
6. All the fingers should touch the ball on the finger pads.
7. Face the target with the shoulders and head, and, if possible, the feet.
8. Follow through by extending the body and arms in the direction of the arc you want the ball to travel.

The *elbows* should be set apart slightly wider than the shoulders. The elbows are prime power sources for the set. This power comes from the extension of the elbows, not, as one might think, the flexion of the wrists. Beginners often use wrist action, which is likely to cause errant sets. The job of the wrists is to control the ball as the extension of the elbows supplies the power.

The power from the elbows must be equal from each elbow or the ball will not fly true. For example, too much power from the right arm will make the ball move to the left of the setter. When the player sets, both arms should be fully extended to ensure an even release.

Side view of contact prior to extension

Arm extension

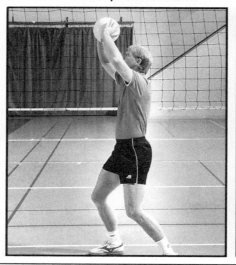
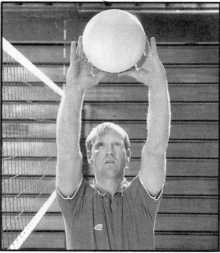

a. hand and arm
follow through,
b. stepping away from
the net to pursue a
pass which is away
from the net

a.

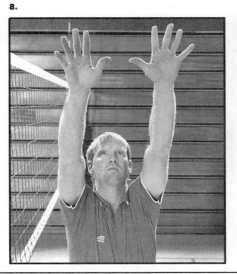

b.

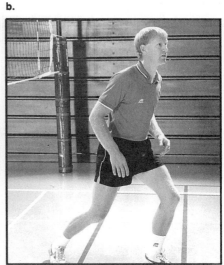

The *shoulders* are essential in aiming the set. They should be aimed directly at the target area. If they are not correctly positioned the ball may be "carried," resulting in a foul. For example, if the target is to the right of the setter and the shoulders are not squared to the target, the left hand will probably stay on the ball longer than the right hand and a "carry" will result. Also, such a set cannot be controlled as well as one in which both arms supply equal impetus to the ball. Not properly squaring the shoulders and feet toward the target area is the most common error in setting.

a. the second step of
pursuit, b. hands
drawn and shaped
with feet squared to
left front attack
position

a.

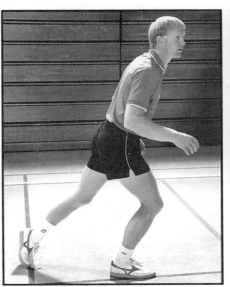

b.

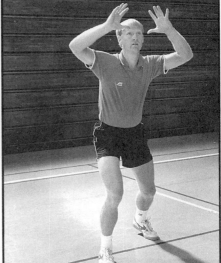

Ball contact prior to extension

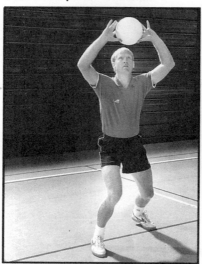

Extension and follow through

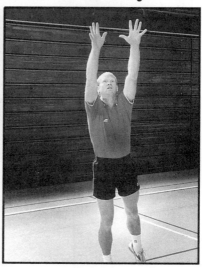

Leg flexion is important, especially for younger players who may not have the upper body strength to set with ball without leg motion. Beginning players are encouraged to use a great deal of knee flexion when setting. This is true whether the set is long and high or short and low. Every setting motion should be uniform, so that opponents cannot predict the kind of set you will make. However, on long sets it is essential to use leg power; in fact, it is not uncommon to see elite players leave their feet as they follow through on long sets. This indicates the considerable amount of leg power they were exerting—even if their legs were not greatly flexed, their ankle muscles helped provide great power.

Some advanced players set the ball with their legs straight, but their upper body strength compensates for this. They do this so that the blockers aren't able to "key" on the amount of knee flexion that they use and thereby tell whether the set will be long or short. If the blocker reads the setter correctly, he or she will be able to anticipate where the ball will go even before it leaves the setter's hands. So at the higher levels of play, perfection and deception are desired.

If at all possible the set should be made with an overhand pass. This requires the setter to bend greatly at the knees. While keeping the hands high, in order to accurately set balls that have been passed low.

Foot positioning is as important as shoulder positioning. For most people the feet should be shoulder width apart, with the right foot forward for better stability. The feet should be pointing at the target area during the setting motion unless the set is an overhead or back set. (Many beginners face the passer rather than the attacker when setting—this is wrong.) However, the feet and shoulders will open toward the passer as the ball is received and then they should rotate back (square) to the target as the set is made. The right foot should be forward to reduce the chance of the set being made too close to the net.

The *contact point* is above the forehead. The setter should watch the ball

Checklist for Common Errors in Setting

1. Getting to the ball too late.
2. Failing to take the ball at the same contact point (above the forehead) each time.
3. Getting the hands up too late.
4. Having the thumbs forward rather than shaped to the ball.
5. Failing to extend to a full reach during the follow through.

through the opening between the thumbs and the index fingers. The ball is taken "on" (above) the forehead.

The *follow through* is very important in accuracy and control. The ball will always go in the direction that it is aimed. If it doesn't go where you desire, you did not aim it there or follow through correctly. The wrists and arms should continue in the direction of the set. Always extend your body to the ball as you follow through.

Varying Types of Sets

Back set:
a. preparing for back set, b. forward weight shift and start of backward extension, c. back set extension, d. back set follow through

Off passes are passes that pull the setter away from the target area. The setter should move past the ball and then turn the body back toward where the attacker will hit. Beginners often merely get to the ball and then have problems setting the ball to the outside. They are likely to throw the ball because they are not squared to the direction of the set.

The setter must get the feet beyond the ball, get set facing the target, and shift his or her weight forward into the set. If the player does not get beyond the ball it will likely fall short of the target.

The *back set* (reverse set) allows the setter to deceive the blockers by using the entire length of the net, no matter which way he or she is facing. The back

a.

b.

c.

d.

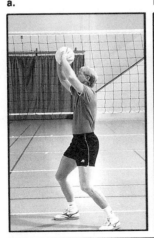
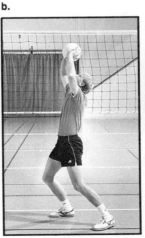
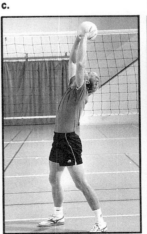
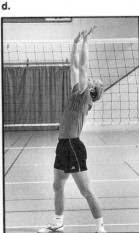

set should look just like the front set so that the blockers are not able to detect where the set will be targeted. However, the back set will be slightly arched and your head will be back so that your arms can direct the ball to the rear and you can watch the flight of the ball during the follow through.

The back set is contacted in the same place as the front set. A common error is that the setter will place the hands lower for a front set and higher for a back set. Another error is running too far under the ball when making the reverse set.

It should be noted that when there is an errant pass, a ball hit high into the net will generally rebound downward, while a ball hit into the low part of the net will usually rebound outward. The exact angle of the ball coming off the net is determined by its speed, the angle at which it hit the net, and the place on the net where it hit.

The setter must note all of the variables listed above and then estimate where the netted ball will go. He or she should then adjust accordingly and drop down as low as possible to play the ball.

The *underhand set* is used as a save technique when it is not possible to set with an overhand pass. It is the same as a bump pass, except that the ball should be placed in an area where the spiker can hit the ball.

The *running set* is a "save" technique, used when a ball is passed so poorly that the setter does not have time to get into position and stop. Even in the running set the setter must square to the target area.

The *jump set* is a valuable technique to use at the intermediate and advanced levels of play. By jump setting, players can increase their effective range and save many balls that might have been unplayable. They may also stop a high pass which might otherwise have traveled over the net before an attacker could hit it. Additionally, jump setting is a way of quickening the attack and allowing the setter to become a potential offensive threat when he or she is in the front row, by occasionally attacking from the jump rather than making the expected set.

When positioning for the jump set, the setter should move as soon as possible to a position one step away from where the ball will come down from the pass.

Jump set
a. start of jump for jump set,
b. drawing the hands for jump set,
c. jumping to the ball with hands shaped,

a.
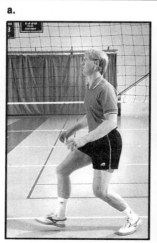

b.
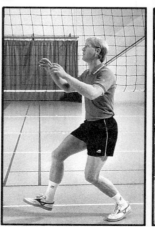

c.
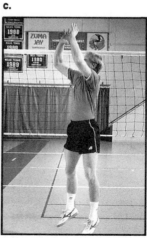

Contact on the jump set

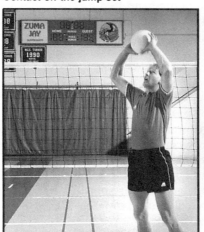

Jump set extension and follow through

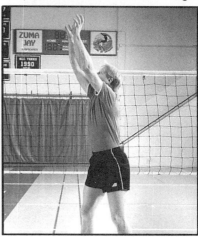

The last step allows the player to collect his or her body for a two-foot takeoff, and also gives the setter time to get his or her hands in the setting position while jumping for the ball.

The jump set requires you to jump as if you were spiking while bringing your hands to the setting position. Time your jump so that the ball is contacted just before the top of the jump. Be sure that your body is facing the direction that you wish the set to travel. If the set is a long one, the follow through of the arms is very important because there can be no additional power from the legs.

A *backward jump set* would be executed using the same techniques as explained for the back set, but is executed at the top of the jump.

A *one-handed jump set* may be used to save a ball that might otherwise go over the net when the pass is too long. Jump as if you were going to spike the

Arm and hand position for one hand set

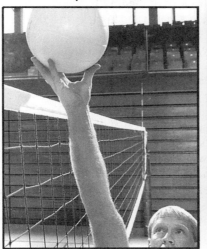

Executing the one hand set

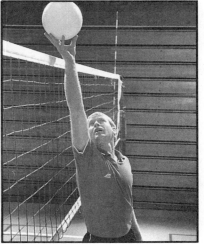

ball, but reach up with the hand closest to the net and, with the fingers spread and stiff and the palm of the hand facing back into your court, make a quick, short contact and direct the ball toward the attacker. The thumb and index finger should be closer together than on a normal set, and the arm and wrist are relatively straight. The power comes from a quick poke or stab of the fingers.

Quick sets are another way of fooling the block. All movements of the setter are kept the same, but the contact is quicker and softer without much follow through. The primary power comes from the hands and fingers.

The quick set is generally short. It should be set far enough away from the net so that the blockers cannot intercept it, and should be high enough so that the attacker can contact it at the highest point possible. The setter should be in a position to see the ball and the attacking arm of the quick hitter.

Once the quick set has been established, a crossing action of two hitters can be played. One attacker can move into the position necessary to play the shorter, "quick" set. A second attacker can move in another direction ready to take the higher "play" set. This can confuse the blockers, who must move to stop the quick set and then move again to stop the play set.

The *play set in a crossing action* should be slightly beyond and behind the quick hitter to allow the play set hitter to move around the quick hitter's approach. The setter again uses a quicker release and allows the ball to be hit as it reaches its peak, or slightly thereafter. The play set timing should remain fairly constant so the hitters will be able to time their approaches the same each time.

In advanced volleyball, *plays* are called that give the players their assignments as to how to cover the court, where to make the pass, the target and height of the set, the attacker, and possibly the direction of the spike.

The *height and placement of the set* in elite volleyball are determined by the play called. The placement may be to a front-court attacker or behind the three meter line to a back-court spiker. In recreational volleyball, the set is usually sufficiently effective if it is two to three feet from the net and about fifteen feet high. This gives the attacker sufficient time to make corrections in the approach and to make the hit.

Considerations for the setter at the more advanced levels are extensive. The setter is the quarterback of the team. It is up to the setter to understand the mood of the team during a match and to evaluate the performance of the attackers. Is one player having a "hot" day? If so, perhaps he or she should receive far more of the sets. By so doing, the setter may instigate a hot streak that may win the game.

The setter must be aware of the opponent's defense. How are the defenders defending a crossing pattern by the attackers?

The setter must also think defensively. When the ball is in the opponent's court, the setter must play the assigned defensive responsibility first and then move to the setting position. Once you have moved to the setting position, let your teammates know that you are there. Call out "I'll set" or "I'm up."

Once the set is made, get into your defensive area of responsibility. As the transition from defense to offense occurs the setter is responsible for the second contact. If the setter is not able to make the second contact, it is essential to call the name of the player who should make the set.

Drills

Beginner

1. Assume the setting position and play with an imaginary ball. Flex the knees as if to get down to low balls. Check the position of arms and hands. Are you holding your arms and hands in the proper position? Are you looking up through the space between your thumbs and fingers for the imaginary ball?
2. Hit the ball against the wall or to a partner. (This can be done sitting, kneeling, squatting, and standing.) In order to get used to setting a low ball, you can allow the ball to bounce from the floor, and then set. Check on your elbow and hand position. When doing the drill standing, make certain that you move your feet properly and that your legs work with the upper body during the setting action.

Incorrect foot position

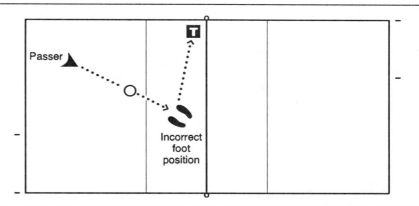

Correct feet

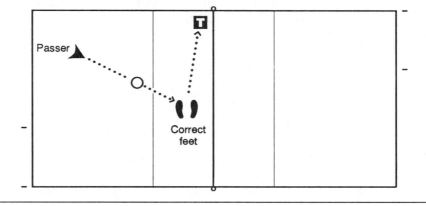

Off pass diagram: past and beyond

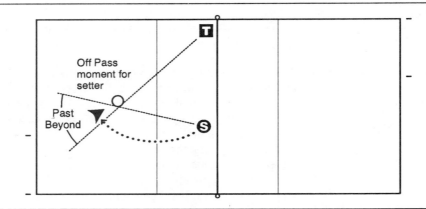

Playset

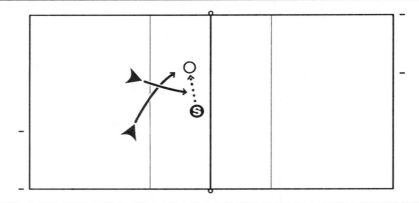

3. With partners, set the ball, turn 360° to the right and set the ball again, then turn 360° to the left and set it once more. Spot the ball as quickly as possible and move your feet to the proper area as you prepare to make contact. Vary the distance between the partners and the height of the sets. Concentrate on the ball and beat the ball to the spot where it will be contacted.

Intermediate

4. With one partner standing on the attack line and another on the back line, have the partners move along the lines while they set. The player on the back line will set diagonally, forcing the attack-line player to move to the spot. The attack-line player then sets straight ahead to the spot where the back-line player has moved. The back-line player sets straight ahead. The attack-line player sets diagonally to the attack-line player. The progression is hit straight twice and then diagonally once.

**Saving ball out
of top of net**

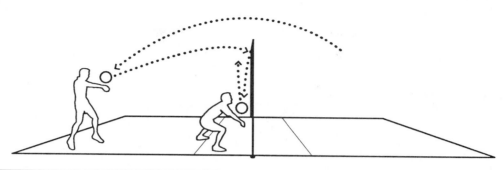

**Saving ball out of
bottom of net**

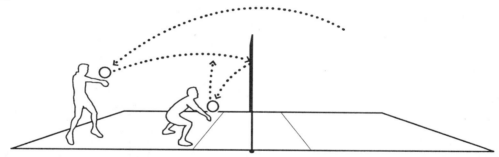

Advanced

5. Your partner or teacher stands in center court (zone 6). The setter (you) moves to the assigned area for the set (zone 3), then executes a front or back set to one of the two spikers positioned on the attack line.
6. The setter starts in left back position (zone 5), and the partner or teacher stands in right back position (zone 1).
7. *Triangle setting*—Passer to setter to target. The target can be a person or an object on the floor.
8. *Four-person with server tossing*—The server tosses or serves the ball over the net, the passer passes to the setter, and the setter sets to the target.
9. *Repetitive setting (setter pressure)*—The coach or passer rapidly makes passes to setter, so that the passes are coming from different directions and at different heights in quick repetition.
10. *Team service*—Receiving for total setter-hitter continuity.
11. Perform the sets in game-related situations with the live passers and attackers.

Endline setting drill

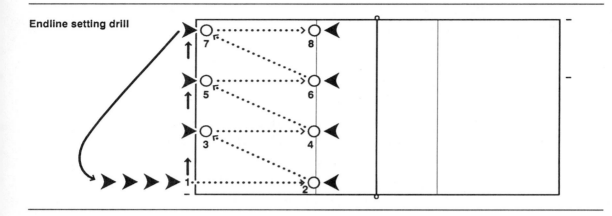

4 person pass set drill

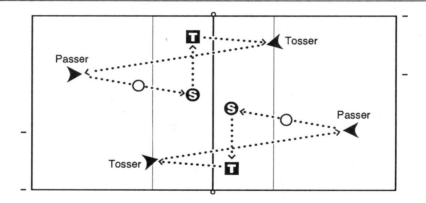

Setter release drill
Setter starts in the right back, goes to the net, sets either front or back and then returns to the right back position.

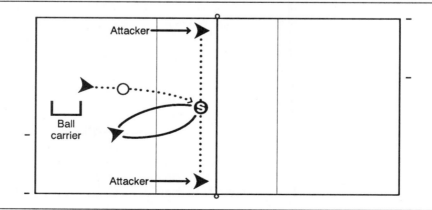

Setter left back release drill
Setter starts in the left back, goes to the net, sets either front or back and then returns to the left back position.

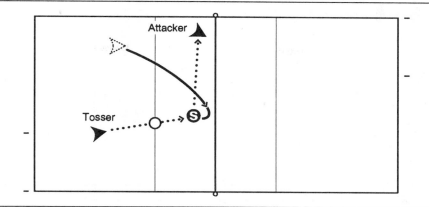

Attacker

Tosser

Checklist for Progression

Beginner level skills:

1. Overhead passing (setting) a tossed ball.
2. Setting a passed ball.

Intermediate skills:

3. Setting "off" passes.
4. Back setting.
5. Underhand setting.
6. Quick setting.

Advanced skills:

7. Running set.
8. Jump set.
9. Play set.
10. One-hand set.
11. Using deception in setting to reduce the blocker's keys.

Triangle setting drill

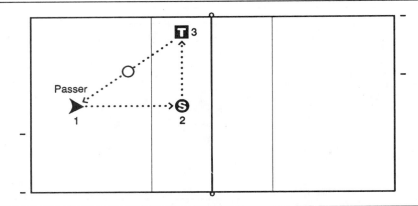

Summary

1. The set is a well controlled overhand pass to an attacker.
2. The set should be made at the correct height and aimed to the exact spot for the attacker to make the kind of attack he or she has planned.
3. In correct setting, the setter must:

   a. Move behind the ball quickly.
   b. Be able to generate sufficient power through a combination of leg and arm extension. (The arm extension is primary.)
   c. Control the ball with the pads of the fingers.

4. Sets may be made from a standing position, a position forward of the setter, or one behind the setter, and can be made while running or jumping.
5. The setter is the quarterback of the volleyball team and must be aware of running the play system and controlling the game.

CHAPTER 6

The Attack

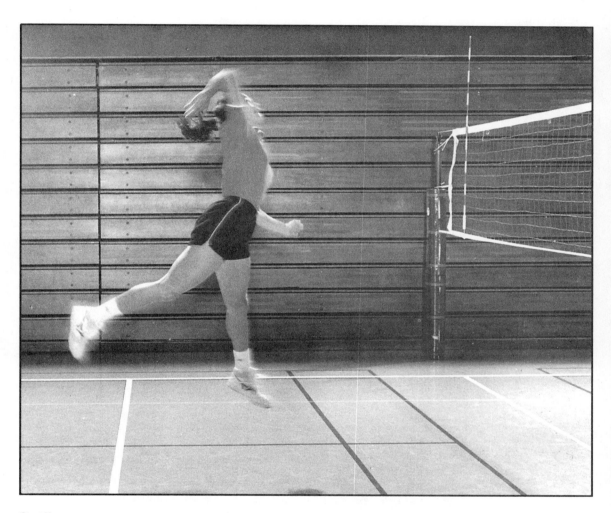

Outline

The attack is the last hit made by the offensive team. It is usually a hard spike, but may be a soft hit just over the blockers (called a "tip" or a "dink,") or a "roll" shot into an open area of the court.

Usually the attack is made on the third contact, but depending on the defensive court coverage or on a variation of offensive strategy, the attack might be on the second or even the first contact of the offensive team. The spike is the most exciting part of a volleyball game.

The Spike

The *spike* is the major offensive weapon of a volleyball team. It is made by the spiker jumping high and contacting the set ball at the maximum height attainable. The spike is then hit hard, usually with top spin, to direct the ball downward into the defenders' court.

The ability to control the body in the air while applying maximum power to the hit is essential to an effective attack. There are three elements of an effective spike: the approach, the jump, and the hit.

The *ready position* is similar in all sports: it allows the player to be able to move in any direction quickly. In the ready position, the player will start with the feet apart about shoulder width or slightly wider. The knees will be flexed. The torso will be bent forward at the waist The weight will be on the balls of the feet. (Some players curl their toes to get the feeling of the weight being forward.) The arms will generally be bent and carried forward. The head will be up.

Once the potential spiker's receiving or defensive responsibilities have been met and the ball has been passed to the setter, the spiker will get to a position about 13 to 14 feet back from the net. The distance from the sideline will depend on the type of attack that has been planned. Beginners and

Initial starting position

First step of the approach

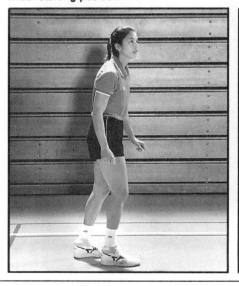
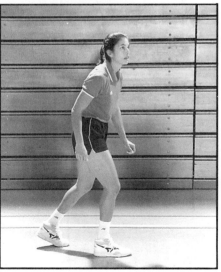

a.   b.   c.

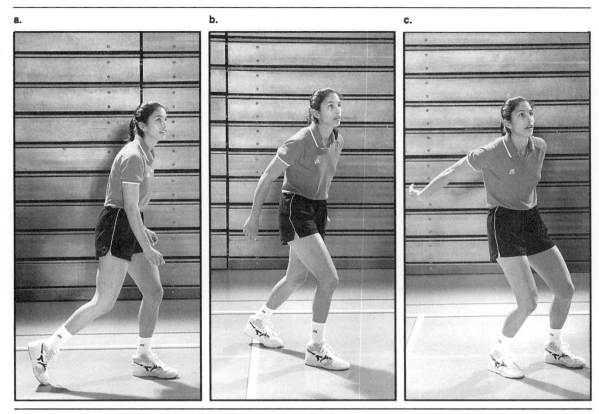

Approach:
a. second step of the
approach, b. third
step of the approach,
c. fast step (gather) of
the approach with
arms back

intermediates are content to merely hit a spike over the net, but advanced players are required to hit to a specific area, often with a special type of hit such as a sharp downward or a deep hit.

The approach can be four, three, or two steps. The number of steps depend on the height of the set and the position of the attacker. The standard four-step approach begins about four or more meters from the net. Starting that far away from the net has three advantages: it allows the spiker to generate horizontal speed that can be transferred into vertical lift on the jump, the spiker can adjust better to a set that is away from the net, and the spiker can adjust more effectively to a set that is made too far right or left of the spiker. (Beginning recreational players will often stand at the net and expect to spike from there. This often contributes to an ineffective spike.)

The standard approach consists of four steps. The first two steps are a timing step and a directional step toward the spot where the set will be spiked. The spiker will take the first step with the leg on the same side as the hitting arm (let's assume this spiker is right-handed, so he or she will take the first step with the right foot). The second step is a rather long one with the left foot. The next right-footed step will be short, as the horizontal drive of the first two steps is transmitted into vertical movement. The last step with the left foot stops the forward movement and prepares for the jump. During the last two steps the knees are flexed and the "gathering" for the jump is completed.

a.

b.

c.

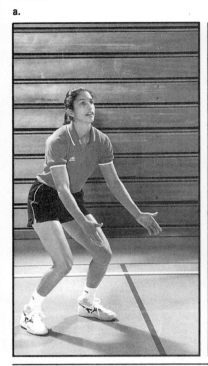
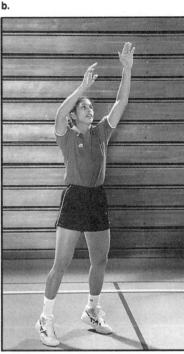
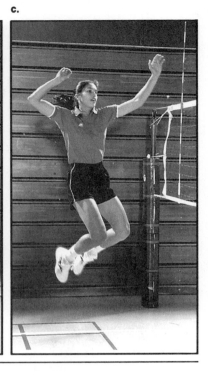

Jump:
a. gather with double arm lift, b. continuation of double arm lift & jump, c. spiking arm drawn back in preparation for arm swing

The *jump* begins during the last two steps of the approach. The arms swing backward and then forward and up as the vertical jump is begun. The power for the jump comes from the front of the thigh (quadriceps muscles), the hips and rear of the thighs (gluteals and hamstrings), with a major thrust from the calf muscle (the gastrocnemius). The arms lead the body upward. The spiking arm is moved backward into the hitting position while the other arm points at the ball to aid the concentration of the spiker. The back is arched to allow the abdominal muscles to stretch and begin the full body snap that delivers the power to the hit.

The abdominal muscles contract, bringing the hips around. Then the shoulders start their forceful movement forward. The legs straighten under the body with the contraction of the abdominals and the hip-flexing muscles. The non-hitting arm is pulled down as the spiking arm moves up and over the ball; these arm movements create a pinwheel effect.

Timing the hit takes practice. The approach should be delayed long enough so that the hitter is able to generate a great deal of speed and power, which will generate an explosive jump. This allows the hitter to reach the ball at the peak of the jump and contact the ball at the highest possible point.

A common error for spikers at all levels is to be over-anxious and start the approach too early. This causes the player to run under the ball and lose power by having to slow down at the end of the approach.

The *hit* is akin to throwing a baseball, but the ball is contacted out in front of the shoulder (8 to 20 inches, 20 to 50 centimeters). The top part of the palm

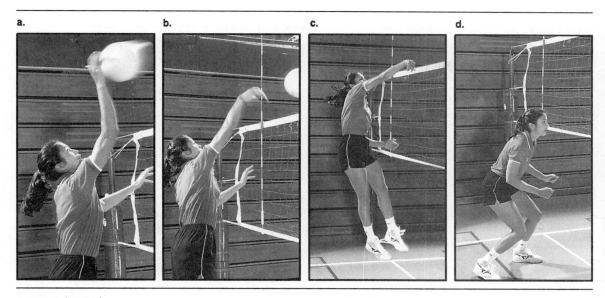

a.   b.   c.   d.

a. arm swing and contact, b. wrist snap and follow through, c. spike follow through, d. post spike cushioned/landing

of the hand, near the fingers, is the major contact point. The fingers then snap over the top of the ball and the hand rotates toward the target area of the court. (It is legal to hit with the fist, but it doesn't give any more power and there is much less control because not as much surface of the ball is being contacted.) The wrist should be loose and allowed to snap freely, as if it were the end of a whip.

The *follow through* will have the shoulders nearly perpendicular to the line of flight to the target. For a right-handed spiker in the right court doing a cross-court spike, the shoulders will be open toward the target. For a down-the-line shot, the shoulders will not be rotated as far around. The force of the hit will have moved the body into a somewhat piked (bent forward at the hips) position. Then the legs will be brought back under the body while preparing to land. The eyes will stay on the ball to see if it has been killed.

The *landing* will be on the toes, with the feet about shoulder-width apart. The attacker will then immediately assume his or her assigned defensive responsibility.

Keep the ball in front as the approach is made. The hitter should be able to see the ball and the block that is forming—with experience and practice this becomes easier to do.

Other Types of Hits

The type of hit will be determined by the hitter's personal arsenal of shots and the way the block has formed. For example, if the block is set inside, the hitter should be able to go down the line. If the middle blocker is late to close the

Side view of ideal arm and hand position   **Back view of hand contact on ball**

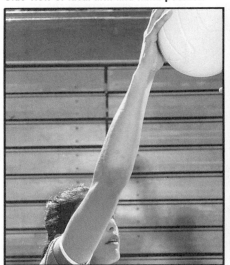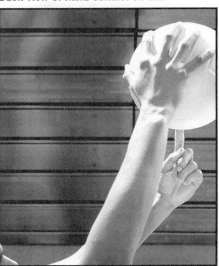

block, the hitter should see this and hit to the seam between the blockers. The hitter may also use a tip or an offspeed shot if an appropriate situation arises.

The *tip shot*, or *dink*, is a change of pace shot. It is a soft shot that may be made when an opening in the defense is spotted beyond the blockers, or when the set is too poor to spike. At more advanced levels it is generally made just over the head of the blockers to an undefended area, or, if there are no blockers, it may be made close to the net. The attacker must know where the defensive weakness is in order to use this skill effectively.

Tipping the ball   **Hitting off the block**   **Wiping the ball off the block**

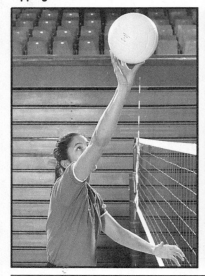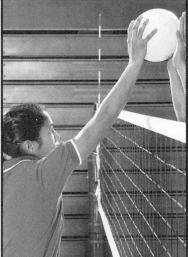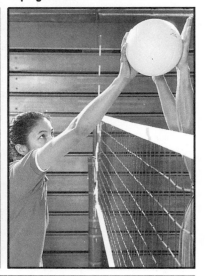

The tip is most effective when made after a fake. The spiker may prepare for the hard hit and then, at the last second, softly touch the ball with the fingertips. The wrist and fingers must be stiff so that the ball leaves the fingers immediately and the player is less likely to be called for carrying the ball.

The *offspeed hit* is much the same as the tip, but the contact is made with the palm of the hand and the motion is the same as for the spike. However, instead of following through after the hit, the arm is slowed or stopped and the wrist snap places the ball over the block and into the open area of the court. This can be a very deceptive play.

Checklist for the Spike

1. Start about three to four meters from the net.
2. The first step will be a timing step with the spiking side leg, and the second step is a directional step toward the target.
3. The last two steps finish with a gathering for the jump.
4. The ball should be hit 8 to 20 inches in front of the spiking arm.
5. The ball is hit with a reach and snap.
6. On landing, the spiker must quickly prepare to play defense.

The *wipeoff* is a shot used when the ball is set too tight to the net to allow the spiker to get it past the block. The approach must be quick and close to the net. The jump must be straight up to avoid going into the net. The ball is taken with the hand open and pushed into the blocker's arms. As the contact is made between the ball and the arms of the blocker, the offensive player turns the wrist outward and pushes the ball off the blocker's arms and out of bounds. Front-row setters can also use this shot on passes made close to the net in which blockers may attack the set.

The quick hit is often the first option in a play system. A good quick hitter can contact the ball before the block is formed. A quick hitter must be fast enough to explode on the ball as the setter releases the set. Generally, the quick hitter will utilize a three-step approach. (Some coaches prefer four steps.) This allows for sufficient momentum to be built up but ensures that the attacker will be in the attack area at the moment that the low set should be hit. Players should be able to use the last two steps (the closing steps) from anywhere on the court. This permits them to step and gather for the jump with only minimal time expended. Unexpected or "off" plays and quick transition plays don't allow the hitter the time to make the preferred four-step approach.

Whatever the number of steps taken in the approach, the hitter should make certain that the set will be hit far enough in front of the body so that he or she can see the block forming. This allows the hitter to determine the type of spike or tip that will be most effective.

Quick hitters will also use an abbreviated arm swing. The backswing will not be extended much past the parallel point of the torso. By reducing the backswing, the armswing can be shortened and quickened.

To make the quick swing, the elbow should come up high and the body rotation should be lessened to enable a quicker snap of the arm. Once the arm is raised, the hitting action should follow immediately. The ball can be contacted as wide as the elbow of the spiking arm or as far inward as the midline of the body. The faster the arm action, the harder the hit. The ball should then be directed with the upper arm and the turn of the wrist.

For *playset hitting* the second hitter delays, then breaks off the quick hitter for a set slightly higher than the quick hitter can reach. Since the set should also be off the net, the playset hitter will "broad jump" more to the spot of the set and will explode into the ball.

By delaying and making a late break, the hitter might cause the block to jump with the quick hitter or be late in forming. This will allow the hitter seams into which to place the ball, as well as helping the hitter to be more explosive and hit the ball harder.

The *back-row attack* has been used more often in recent years to offset the larger and stronger blockers. The back-row attack allows the offense to incorporate virtually any hitter, whether in the front row or back row, into offense.

One of the major benefits of the back row hit is the fact that since the ball is contacted farther off the net, the attack angles are less acute and the ball becomes harder to block. A good hitter will develop both a cross-court and a down-the-line hit, which enable him or her to attack a poorly formed or a drifting block.

The approach will be from two or three meters behind the three-meter line, but instead of jumping straight up on the last steps the hitter will broad jump over the three-meter line. (As long as the attacker takes off from behind the line, the ball can be hit forward of the line.) The placement of the set will be determined by the spiker's jumping and hitting ability. The placement should permit the hitter to spike the ball at the peak of the jump.

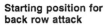
Starting position for back row attack

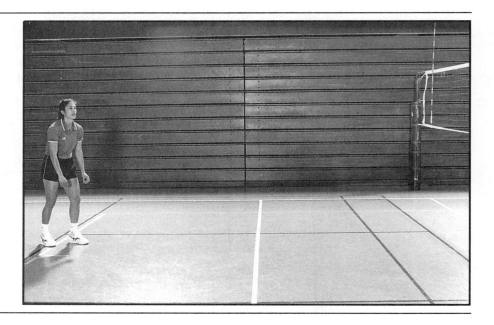

First step of approach for back row attack

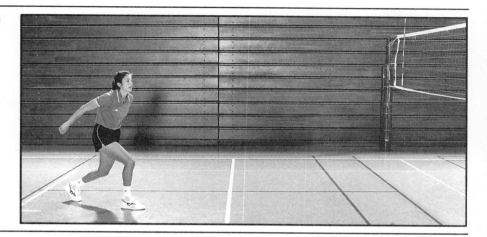

Second step of approach for back row attack

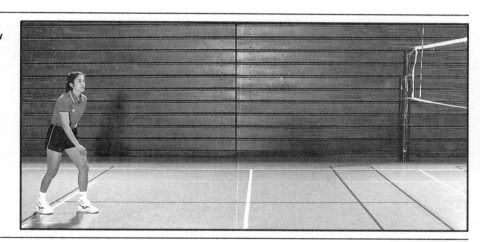

Gather with arms back

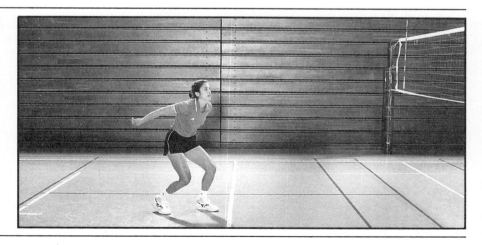

Double arm lift in preparation for broad jump

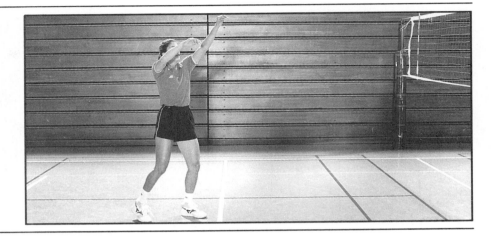

Broad jump with arm in spiking position

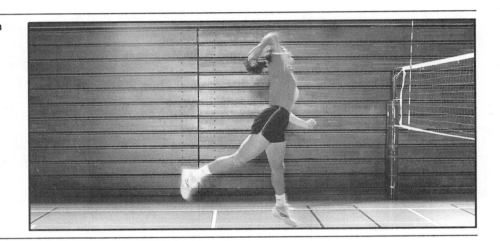

Arm moving just prior to contact

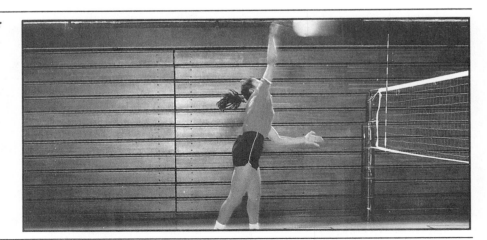

Swing-hitter movement

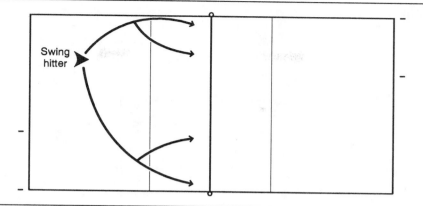

Swing hitting is a term brought into use in recent years to describe the activity of an attacker who can move (swing) from one area of the court to another to spike. This movement can confuse the blockers.

A swing-hitting player may be lined up in the left forecourt and then swing to the right forecourt to spike. This type of movement keeps the defense off balance and makes it difficult for them to commit their blockers by watching only the potential hitters who are near the set.

The *one-foot attack* has become an effective play to beat or move large blockers by creating quick movement laterally along the net. The player will move along the net and jump off of one foot to attempt to drive past where the blockers set up. Normally right-handed hitters break to the right and left-handed hitters to the left.

The *lob* is a shot directed over the opposing players into an open area. It is used in the hope that it will force the defenders into the back court and bring about a poor pass. The lob is contacted from behind and below the ball.

 Checklist of Common Errors in Spiking

1. Having the hand contact the underside of the ball rather than behind and on top of the ball.
2. Lifting with only one arm during the jump.
3. Hitting with a closed hand.
4. Overrunning the set so that the ball is behind, rather than in front of, the hitter.
5. Not having the non-spiking shoulder facing the net.
6. Keeping the elbow too low.

Drills

1. *Outside in hitting*—The attacker starts three meters from the net and outside the sideline.

Outside-in hitting

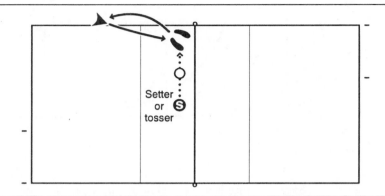

2. *Four-way step close*—A two-step drill in which the attacker goes forward, right, left, and back, hitting a tossed ball after each movement.

4-way step close
Player uses only
2 steps (step close)
to spike balls that
are tossed one at a
time to the four
areas shown.

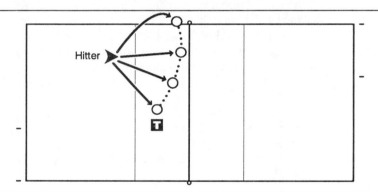

3. *Multiple-area deep hitting*—The attacker hits the ball to designated areas of the court.

Court placement

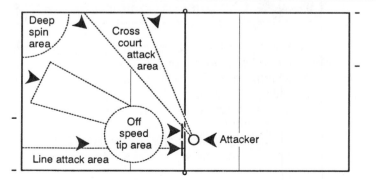

**Multiple area
deep hitting**

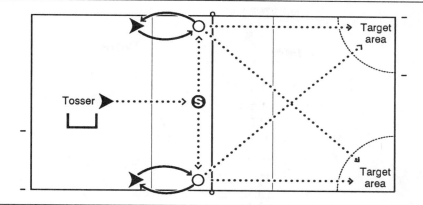

4. *Power and vision*—The teacher stands on a box on one side of the net and moves his or her arms right or left in a blocking motion. The attacker, who is on the other side of the net, hits a set or tossed ball opposite the direction to which the teacher is moving his or her arms.

Power and vision
Attacker tries to
hit the ball away
from the blocker.

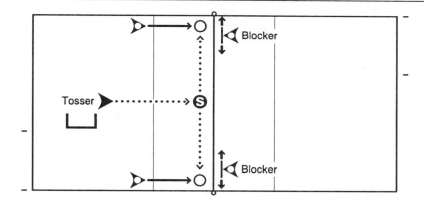

Summary

1. The attack is the last hit made by the offensive team.
2. Generally, the most effective hit is a spike.
3. The spiker generally starts the approach from three to four meters back from the net.
4. There are several types of spikes: the playset hit, the quick hit, the backcourt hit.
5. Other types of attack hits are: the tip or dink, the wipeoff, and the offspeed.

Checklist for Progression

Beginner:

1. Jump and swing.
2. Approach.
3. Arm lift and arm snap.

Intermediate:

4. Tip shot.
5. Offspeed or roll shot.
6. Ability to hit into different areas of the court.

Advanced:

7. Wipeoff.
8. Quick hit.
9. Playset hit.
10. Back-row attack.
11. Swing hitting.
12. One-foot attack.

The Serve

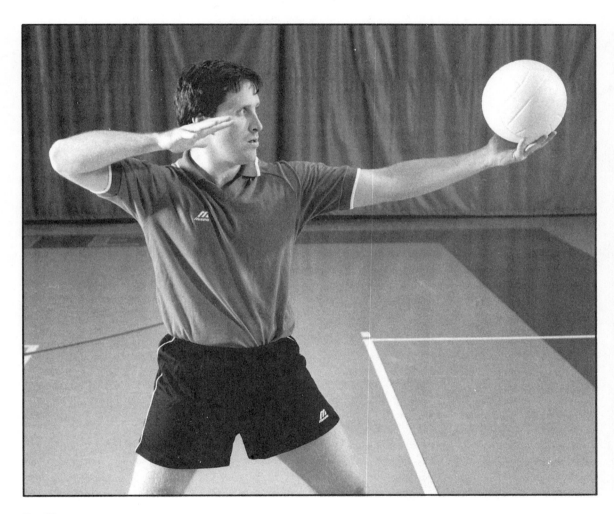

Outline

The serve is obviously an integral part of a volleyball match. A highly effective serve will score an outright winner—an ace. Even if it is not an outright winner, a serve can still put the opponents in a weaker position by forcing an errant pass and possibly a weak set. The best method of derailing a potent offense is to deliver a tough serve and force them into a slower or less desired option of attack.

There are several types of serves. Top players may master a number of them, but few players master them all. As a beginner, the most important factors in serving are speed and accuracy. The first goal is to get the ball into the court with speed; the next concern is to maneuver the ball to the defense's weakness.

The rules require that the server remain behind the end line until the ball is contacted. The server must serve the ball from within three meters of the right sideline. Should the server serve from too wide a position or step on the line before the ball leaves his or her hand, it would be a fault and the serve would be lost.

 Checklist for the Serve

1. Starting position.
2. Backswing.
3. Toss.
4. Stride.
5. Hit.
6. Follow through.

The Underhand Serve

The *underhand serve* can be extremely effective at the beginning level. Since it is easy to learn, it has a greater chance of achieving the accuracy rate desired by beginning-level players.

The *stance* begins by facing the target and then taking a stride forward with the non-serving side leg. The feet will be about shoulder-width apart. The forward foot should face the direction of the serve, and the knees should be slightly flexed. The foot cannot touch the line. Most players serve from two to ten feet behind the back line.

The *serving action* starts with the ball in the non-serving hand (left hand for right-handed servers). It is held with the palm up, in front and outside of the serving-side hip. The ball is lifted straight up just a few inches from the non-serving hand. (Hitting directly from the hand is illegal.)

The hitting arm swings backwards as the weight is shifted to the rear foot and the shoulders turn away from the net with the backswing. The weight

**Starting posture for
underhand serve**

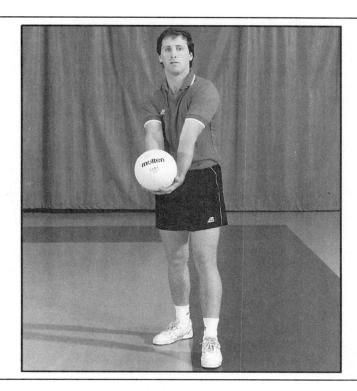

then shifts forward and the hips and shoulders rotate toward the target. The arm swings forward and contacts the ball with the heel of the hand and a stiff wrist or a fist. (The stiff wrist limits the amount of spin on the ball.) The ball is contacted below the center. Keep your eyes on the ball throughout the serve.

The arm follows through toward the target and the server moves into the court, ready to take up the assigned defensive position.

Serving arm drawn back   **Ball lift and stride**   **Arm swing prior to contact**   **Contacting the ball**

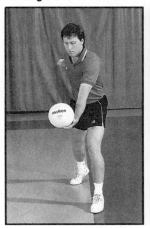 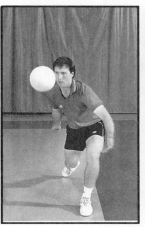 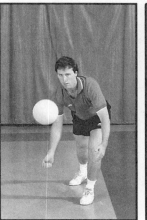 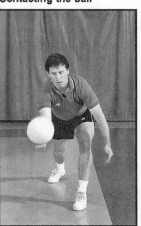

Side view of stride

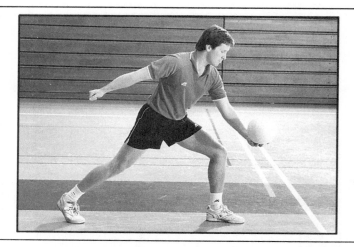

A high underhand serve may be quite difficult for the receivers to play. Indoors, the ball may move unexpectedly because of the buildup of air pressure under the ball. Outdoors, the ball may be carried by the wind, which will alter the ball's trajectory and make it hard to handle. If it is sunny and the opponents are facing the sun, the ball may be played so that it is hidden in the sunlight.

The Overhand Serve

There are several types of overhand serves, among them floaters, spins, and jumps. Each has a unique technical form.

The *starting position* is facing the net with the feet shoulder-width apart and positioned under the shoulders. The left foot (for right-handed servers) will be forward in a comfortable stance. The ball is held in both hands at about chest to shoulder height. The non-serving hand is under the ball while the serving hand rests on top.

Starting posture for float serve

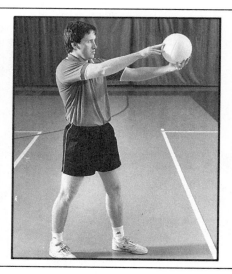

Backswing:
a. drawing the serving elbow and hand back,
b. start of arm swing with elbow lead and ball placement

a.

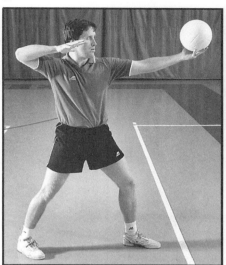

b.

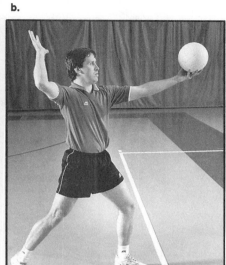

The *backswing* is like a catcher's throw rather than a full-arm swing. The elbow is drawn back and remains above the shoulder. As the arm is moving back, the shoulder and hips rotate away from the net. At or near the end of this action, the ball is lifted up about two feet high and about one to one and one-half feet in front of the hitting shoulder. A low, accurate toss helps the serve to be efficient.

The *stride* with the non-hitting side leg starts the serving action. As the server steps forward, the weight is shifted to the forward foot. The hips and shoulders turn toward the net. The hitting arm closely follows in a forward action.

Arm position just prior to contact

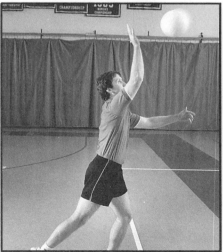

Post ball contact showing open firm hand

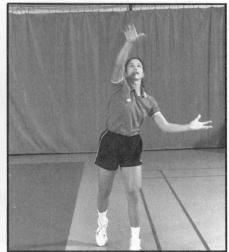

Two-step serve:
a. second and final
step of two step
serve, b. side view of
two step float serve
showing first of two
steps

a.

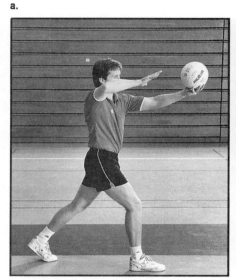

b.

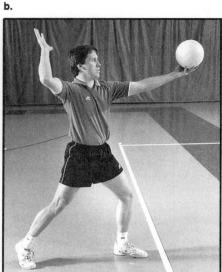

The *elbow leads the hand and arm* as the hitting arm comes forward. The shoulder comes forward, then the elbow extends, then the wrist follows through. The ball is contacted just above head height and in front of the hitting shoulder.

The wrist remains stiff and the hand is open to offer the largest surface area possible. The wrist should not turn but instead should direct the hand toward the serving target.

The *two-count toss* is often valuable for beginners because it can give them more power. In this movement, the striking-side leg steps forward (right leg for right-handed server), and the striking hand is drawn back as the first step is made.

Initial posture for top spin serve

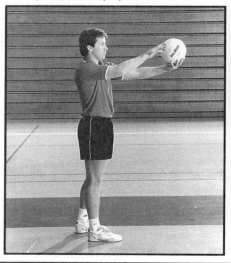

Ball lift and back arch

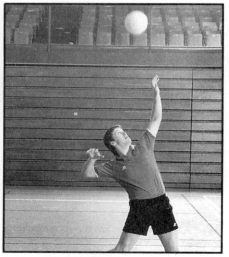

Arm extension and contact point, snapping the wrist to put top spin on ball

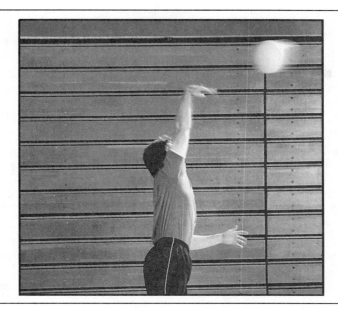

The toss is made when the second step is started. As the weight is transferred to the non-striking side foot (left foot for right-handers), the arm moves forward, striking the ball.

The *hand contacts the ball* on the palm. The trajectory of the ball should be nearly flat. A high-trajectory overhand serve is no more effective than an underhand serve.

The *follow through* is toward the target. As the arm follows through, the player moves into the court to take up the assigned defensive position.

The Float Serve

The *float serve* is the most commonly used serve at the elite levels of play in the United States. It is a non-spinning ball that will move with the existing air currents. It begins with the same stance as the underhand serve. The player will generally take a position from two to ten feet behind the back line. The non-serving leg is forward and the feet are about shoulder-width apart.

The ball is held with the palm up, about chest level or higher. Because the ball's valve makes that area of the ball heavier, the ball may drift to the side of the valve. This theory has been advanced for years but it has not been proven.

The ball is lifted with the non-serving hand from an area in front of the hitting shoulder. It should be two to three feet high and just in front of the hitting-side shoulder. The eyes remain on the ball throughout the serve.

The hitting arm swings back as the weight is shifted to the rear foot. The weight then is moved forward as first the hips then the shoulders swing through. The arm follows as in a baseball throw. The ball is contacted with an open hand in the middle of the back of the ball. The contact point is slightly higher than the head. The primary impact is with the heel of the hand. The wrist is locked.

Checklist for the Floater Serve

1. Stand back from the back line, facing the court.
2. Toss the ball in front of the hitting shoulder, two to three feet high, with no spin.
3. Hit into the back of the ball.
4. Keep the hand open and wrist solid.
5. Limit the follow through.
6. After making the serve, get back into a defensive position.

There is little follow through because the ball is punched. (Note, however, that a player who is not very strong may have to follow through.) After making the shot, the player moves into the court to play defense.

A hard float serve is struck hard on the middle of the ball. It moves faster and is lower than the regular float serve.

The Top-Spin Serve

The *top-spin serve* is effective because it allows for a fairly powerful serve with relative accuracy. With the top-spin, the server takes a position much the same as a tennis serve. The ball is tossed up as the hitting shoulder rotates away from the ball.

The ball is tossed higher than for a floater, to allow the player to hit the underside of the ball (about 30° below the center of the back of the ball) and then drive the hand over the top of the ball with a snap of the wrist.

As a variation the hand can follow through to either side of the ball, causing a side spin. This can be especially effective when playing outside with a crosswind. The ball can be spun so that the wind's role in pushing the ball is greatly increased.

The Jump Serve

The *jump serve* can be highly effective, but it is rather risky. Because of all the variables involved (the run, jump, and wrist action), the accuracy is reduced.

The start of the serve is the same as an approach for a spike. For a right-handed server, the four-step approach would be right, left, step, close, jump. The three-step approach would start with the left leg. The toss is made prior to the "step, close" portion of the approach, so that the ball can be contacted at the peak of the jump and slightly ahead of the body. The toss can be made with one or two hands.

As with the spike, the hand and wrist will snap over the top to achieve power and control. Most players will toss the ball so that their momentum will actually carry them over the end line of the court. This is legal as long as the ball is contacted prior to landing. The momentum of the approach and the jump is transferred to the ball, which greatly increases the arm power and ball speed.

Jump serve:
a. initial posture for
jump serve, b. first
step of approach,
c. ball placement (lift)
and start of jump
d. full lift and jump,
just prior to contact
e. post contact posi-
tion with follow
through (see c , d , e
below)

a.

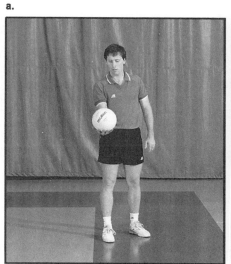

b.

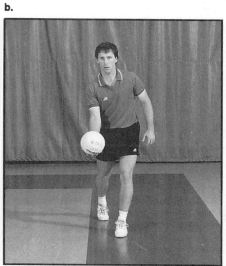

As with the top-spin serve, the action of the wrist can cause the ball to spin sideways, making it an even tougher serve. The speed and spin of the ball make it very difficult to play at the lower levels of volleyball, but at the elite level the skill of the passers reduces the serve's effectiveness because they can predict where the ball will land. The hard-spinning serves give a true trajectory as opposed to the floater serve, which is unpredictable in the direction it will move. In higher levels of competition, speed and accuracy must be increased to remain effective.

c.

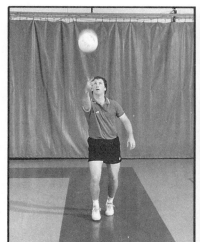

d.

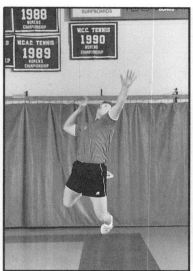

e.

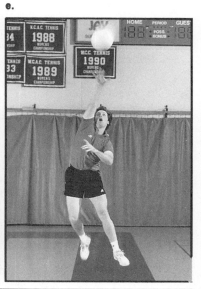

Other Considerations

The *serving areas* (zones 1 through 6) may be targeted by the coach in high levels of play. At lower levels, the players need merely be aware that they should have a specific target to which to serve. Using the whole court as the target is appropriate only for the very beginning-level player.

Serving area

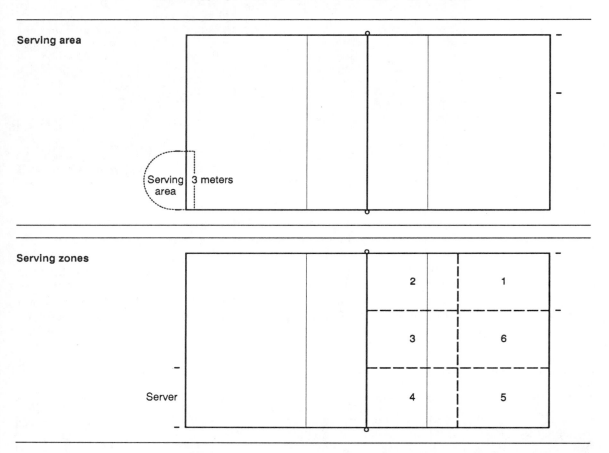

Serving zones

Varying the trajectories is another way to complicate the opponents' passing. By beginning with high, deep serves to force the passers to align deeper into their court, the server can open up the front area for shorter-diving top-spin serves.

It is important that the passers don't get into a rhythm of playing balls of the same speed and trajectory. The good server will vary the serves to prevent the receivers from getting into that groove.

Concentration and *ritual* are the final considerations for serving. By developing a ritual or procedure for use prior to each serve, the server can prepare his or her body for the relatively simple motor action of the serve. This practice also aids in relaxation and concentration. A simple ritual might be to simply bounce the ball once or twice; a more complicated ritual might be to close the eyes, take three deep breaths to relax, then put the middle finger of the tossing hand on the valve.

High trajectory serve

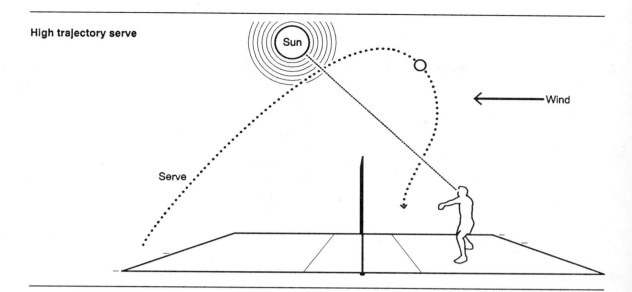

Checklist for the Server's Priorities

1. Be consistent and get nearly every serve into the opposite court.
2. Serve to the proper target area—the weak player or the vulnerable area (rear corners or seams between players).
3. Higher-level players should do something special to the serve: increased speed, a tricky spin, or a lack of spin.

Strategies for Serving

- Always know your target area and the type of serve you want to hit before beginning your service action.
- Find out before the game which of your opponents is the weakest serve returner, or quickly discern who it is as you play. A substitute who has just entered the game may be a good target because he or she may not be warmed up.
- The weakest areas in a defense usually are the deep corners, the sidelines, the short middle area, and the seams between the players.
- Sometimes serve into the setter's path as he or she moves from the back court to the forecourt.
- Vary the targets as the opponents adjust their serve receive.
- The primary concern of the server is to get the ball over the net and in play.

Checklist of Common Errors in Serving

1. Having a problem in timing the serving action, such as bringing the arm through before the weight has shifted or the hips have turned. People who have not had much experience in throwing will often make this type of error.
2. Taking too short a stride to get an effective weight shift.
3. Bringing the arm through too low in the forward swing.
4. Not serving fast enough (arm action too slow).
5. Having the wrist too loose when contacting the ball.
6. Failing to hit the center of the ball.

Drills

Serving practices should be distributed throughout the practice session, rather than encompassing one long segment during the practice.

1. *Partner serving*—Servers at each end of the court serve into the opposite court.

Partner serving

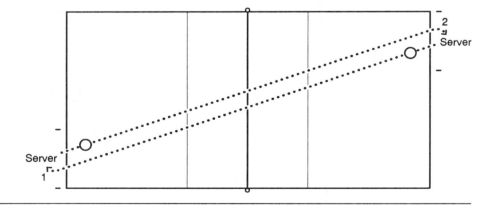

2. *Target serving*—Set up targets, people, or "Bozos" (the air-filled, bottom-weighted, pop-up, simulated clowns). Serve to hit the target.
3. *Four–two triangle serving*—One server versus two passers and a setter. The passers get one point if they make four consecutive good passes. The server gets a point if he or she makes two good serves that cannot be played.

Target serving

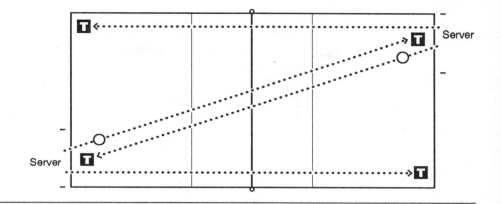

4 versus 2 triangle serving
To score a point the passer must pass four perfect passes consecutively. The server scores when the passer fails to pass perfectly two consecutive times. The scoring criteria can be adjusted to fit the level of play.

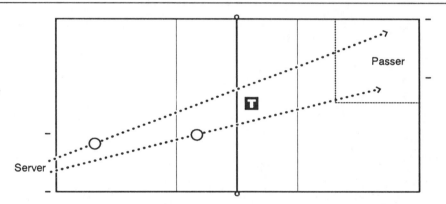

4. *"Elastic" serving*—Serving between the top of the net and a single line of elastic 2, 3 or 4 feet above the net.

Checklist for Progression

Beginner:
1. Underhand serve.
2. Overhand serve.

Intermediate:
3. Float serve.
4. Hard float serve.
5. Top-spin serve.

Advanced:
6. Jump serve.

Summary

1. When learning to serve, do not sacrifice speed for accuracy.
2. The elbow should be kept high while serving.
3. There are several types of serves: underhand, standard overhand, spin serves, floaters, and jump serves.
4. The server should have a clear idea as to where to serve by identifying the weak area of the defense or the weak player in the defense.

CHAPTER 8

Blocking

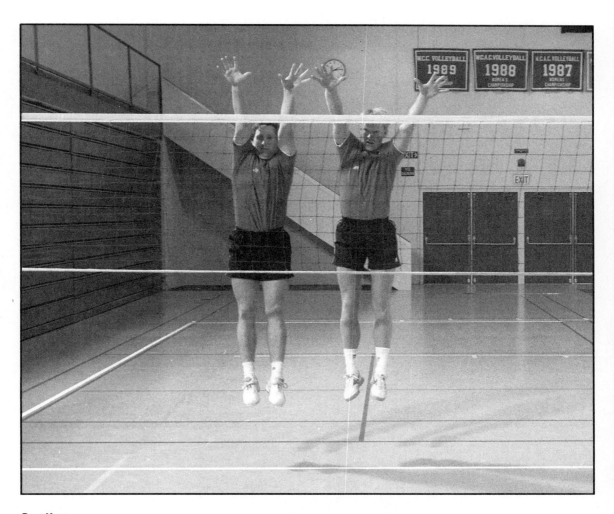

Outline

Introduction

Blocking is a key defensive tactic in volleyball—it is the first line of defense against an attack. Properly executed, it eliminates or reduces the effectiveness of the attack. However, at the very beginning level of play, it is not too important because there are not many spikes to block. Also, unless a player can reach over the net, he or she should not block. Such a player will be more effective in court coverage than by jumping up next to the net.

The most important concept to remember when blocking is that the ball must be intercepted on the opponent's side of the net. Because of this requirement, blocking is a very complex skill that must be constantly practiced (as with any other complex skill).

Blocking is one of the most challenging skills to learn because it is difficult to break it up into its many parts and practice each part individually. The best way to learn to block is to execute the entire movement at 100 percent effort—physically and mentally.

The block can be made by one, two, or three players. (The most common block is the two-person block.) For years the teaching and coaching emphasis has been on all aspects of offense, individual defense, and ball control; blocking techniques and tactics have been overlooked. And of the information available on blocking, most is concerned only with technique. This chapter will address both concerns.

The *starting position* is at arm's length from the net. The knees will be slightly flexed and the hands at head height or higher in a ready position. (The better the pass, the higher the hands.) The eyes watch the ball, the setter, and the potential hitters in order to anticipate where the spike is likely to occur.

The two outside blockers are within three steps from their nearest sidelines and at least one meter from the middle blocker. This enables the middle blocker on an outside set to take a big step and not interfere with the outside blocker.

Initial starting position

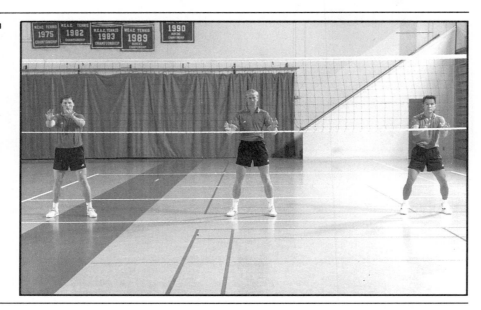

Side view of starting posture showing measure

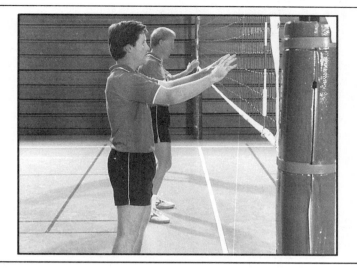

The Eye-Contact Sequence

The blockers watch the passed ball to the apex of its flight. If the ball is passed over the net, the blocker hitting it should do so hard. If the pass is good, the blocker should prepare to block by reading the setter and the setter's release. (It is desirable for the blockers to observe the attacker out of their peripheral vision, but their main visual focus should be on the setter and the setter's release.) All sets can be judged by the initial speed of the ball. The eye contact sequence can be reduced to "ball-setter, ball-hitter."

Reading the setter is a way to anticipate the height and direction of the set. It allows the blocker to move quickly to the area of the attack.

- A setter with low hand position will often set low and to the outside.
- A shoulder dropped toward the net may tip off a short set to the middle.

Eye contact sequence starts by watching setter.

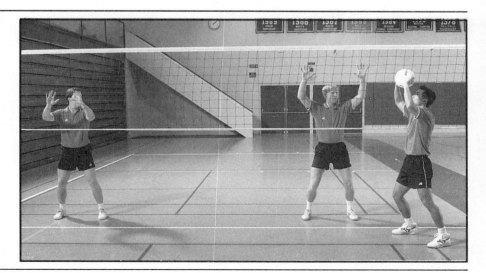

Blocker takes second step and watches hitter

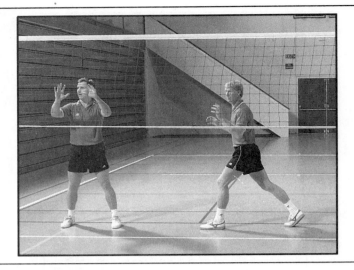

- A setter moving farther under the ball may be tipping off a back set.
- A full extension of the knees is likely to indicate a high set.
- The direction of the follow through indicates the direction of the set.

Reading the attacker is the next part of the eye-contact sequence. Once the blocker has identified where the set is going, his or her focus changes from the ball to the attacker. The longer the blocker looks at the attacker, the more the blocker is able to observe. The blocker's reaction is slowed if the look is only momentary. The blocker should "read up" the hitter by identifying the attacker's point of origin and the attacker's line of approach, and culminate with a visual fix on the attacker's hitting shoulder and hitting arm. The final point of focus is watching the hitter contacting the ball.

Blocker watches hitter and penetrates the net

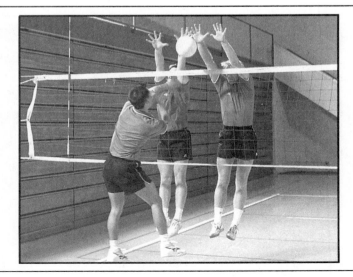

Footwork

There are two types of footwork patterns in blocking, the shuffle and the crossover. The shuffle is used to cover short distances up to one or two meters. The crossover is used to cover more ground in setting up for a block. Whichever pattern is used, the feet must move into the proper position because the block is set with the feet, and then the ball is blocked with the hands.

The *shuffle* is similar to the basketball defensive slide action, so it is easily learned by those who have played basketball. In the shuffle the leg nearest the target area is moved first; the trailing leg is then closed. The shuffle may be a series of two-step (step and close) movements. If these two steps get the blocker to the point of attack, he or she prepares to jump as the trailing leg closes to the lead leg.

Shuffle step—stuffing ball to floor

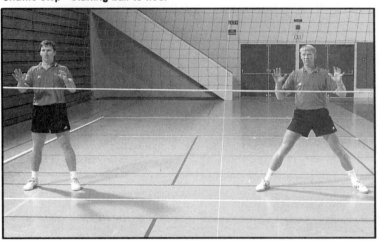

Feet together (gather)

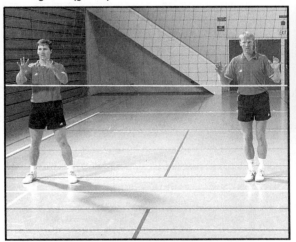

Second shuffle

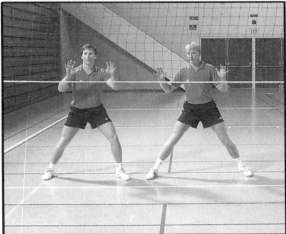

Gather for blocking jump

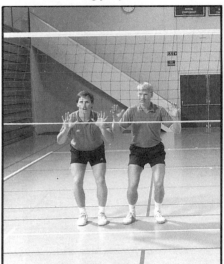

Blocking jump

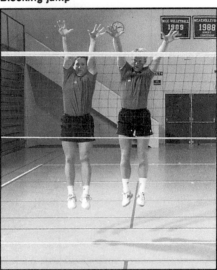

The *crossover* starts with a long lead step (the leg nearest the target), and then the trailing leg crosses over in front of the leading leg—gaining the required distance. Then the lead leg closes and the blocker prepares to jump. This is normally a three-step movement, but it can be a five-step movement if the target area is a long way from the blocker. Hence the crossover is similar to turning and running to the point of attack.

The problem with the crossover is that when the blocker finally arrives at the place where the block will occur, he or she must reorient to the net. This is done by facing the net, placing the shoulders square to the net, and positioning oneself the proper distance away from it—about arm's length. The blocker should always bend at the knees, not at the waist.

 ## Checklist for Blocking

1. Be in the ready position at arm's distance from the net.
2. Watch the ball as it is set.
3. Move to where the ball will be hit.
4. Watch the hitter as you move and jump.
5. Jump just after the hitter jumps.
6. Extend the arms over the net (penetrate and seal) as you jump.
7. Reach as far into your opponent's court as possible. The ball must be intercepted on the opponent's side of the net.
8. Watch the hitter's arm and shoulder as the ball is contacted.
9. Ball-setter, ball-hitter.

The jump of the blocker occurs just after the attacker jumps. The blocker will jump as high as possible while moving the arms over and across the net. The movement is not "jump up then put your arms over the net;" the proper movement is "jump up while simultaneously sliding your arms across the net." This seals the net by not allowing space between the arms and the net in which the ball can go under the blocker's arms.

Armwork

Net penetration (extending the arms over the net) is essential for making an effective block. The blockers must penetrate the opponents' air space as deeply as possible without touching the net. The angle of the arms should direct a blocked ball downward toward the center of the opponent's court.

The blockers should be able to perceive the backs of their hands in their peripheral vision field as they watch the attacker strike the ball. This will help to ensure that the hands are over the net, rather than merely above the net. It also helps the blocker to put his or her hands either on the ball or in the area in which the ball may travel.

The *arm position* will be fully extended with the fingers spread, the thumbs nearly touching, and the little fingers turned outward as far as possible. The fingers should be spread to take up as much area as possible.

Good blockers block balls with their hands, not their arms. The outside blockers should cover the attacker's hitting arm to take away the straight spike, and the middle blocker should take away the attacker's crosscourt shot.

As soon as the spike has occurred or the block has been made, the arms are quickly brought back to the blocker's side of the net.

Back view of blocking form

Side view of net penetration

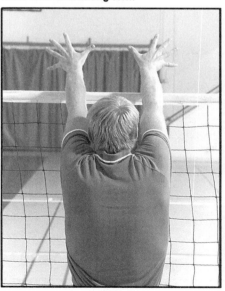

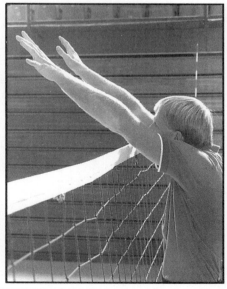

Checklist of Common Errors in Blocking

1. Attempting to block when you are unable to reach over the top of the net.
2. Staying with the set ball too long rather than reading the attacker.
3. Having your body too close to the net, resulting in a netting error and no penetration.
4. Having your arms straight up in the air.
5. Waving your arms excessively.

Blocking Tactics

Blocking systems can be categorized as the read or the commit-stack. In the read system, all blockers *read* the setter and then react to the set. The blocker's weight distribution is neutral and the blocker does not move until the direction of the set is read.

Stack blocking left side set

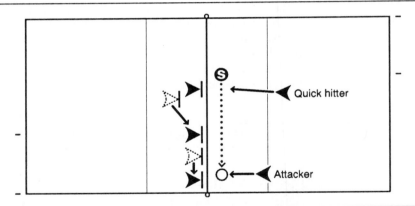

Read blocking for a right side attacker

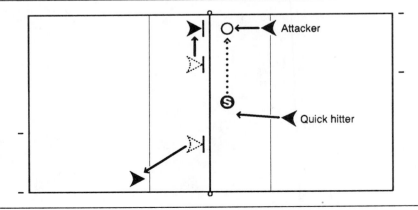

In the *commit-stack* scheme, one blocker is aligned behind the other in a stack. The first blocker (the commit blocker) takes out the quick hitter and tries to block the quick attack if it should come. This is the first blocker's sole responsibility.

The stack blocker aligns behind the commit blocker and then breaks right or left, depending on the set or the movement of the playset hitter. The stack blocker can read the setter or follow a designated hitter.

**Stack blocking
left side set**

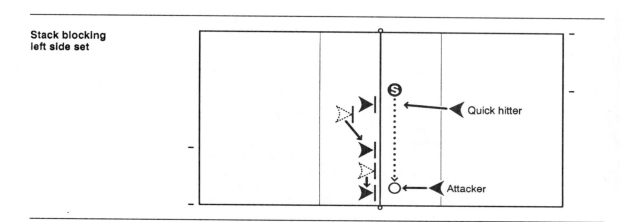

**Stack blocking
right side set**

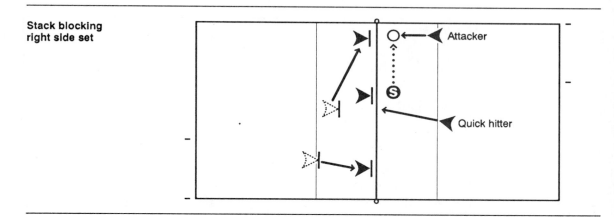

Drills

1. *Blocking while standing*—This is done by lowering the net to about four and one-half to five feet or by having the players stand on a table. An attacker on the opposite side of the net tosses the ball just above the net on his or her side of the net. The blocker stuffs the ball down to the floor while remaining standing. Each player should stuff about ten balls.
2. *Offspeed hit to target*—This is performed with the same lowered net or table. A hitter hits an offspeed (slowed up) spike to a predetermined spot. The blocker, knowing the direction of the hit, stuffs the ball to the floor.

3. *Penetrate and return*—This is learned by using the same props as above (low net or table). One player tosses the ball easily, just above the net. The blocker reaches over the net, catches the ball, and returns the arms quickly to his or her side of the net.

4. *Hand position*—This is reinforced by using the same low net or two tables (one for the teacher/coach and one for the two blockers). The teacher hits into the block while watching the hand position of the blockers. The outside blocker must have his or her hand turned in to stop the "wipe-off" shot.

5. *See the attacker*—A coach or teacher stands behind the blocker and tosses a set over the blocker and the net to an attacker. The blocker fronts the attacker and attempts to block every spike.

6. *Three blockers vs. two attackers*—Middle blocker reads the set and immediately goes to point of attack. The attackers are outside on both sides.

7. *4–1–5 offense*—Three blockers work against three hitters using a 4–1–5 offense only. (4–1–5 offense: A ball is set to zone 4, a 51 set, or a 95 set. See Chapter 10 on team offense for an explanation of this numbering system.)

8. *Reading and reacting*—Three blockers block against any offense. Emphasize reading the setter and reacting to the set.

9. *Block and recover*—This is drilled by having the teacher, who is standing on a table, use two balls. One ball is hit into the block and then the second ball is tossed near the net, to force the blockers to recover from the block and play the ball, which is now on their side of the net.

 Checklist for Progression

Beginners:
1. Eye contact.
2. Block jump.

Intermediate:
3. Footwork pattern.
4. Arm movement.

Advanced
5. Read, commit-stack techniques.
6. Read attacker's approach and armswing.

Summary

1. The block is one of the most difficult skills to master in volleyball.
2. The blocker should constantly measure the distance to the net.
3. The blocker must see the ball as it is passed, set, and then move toward the area of the attack.
4. The blocker will jump while extending the arms over the net, to seal and penetrate the opponent's area.
5. The blocker must watch the attacker contact the ball.
6. The ball should be blocked to the center of the court, if possible.
7. There are two blocking schemes, the read and the commit-stack.

CHAPTER 9

Individual Defense

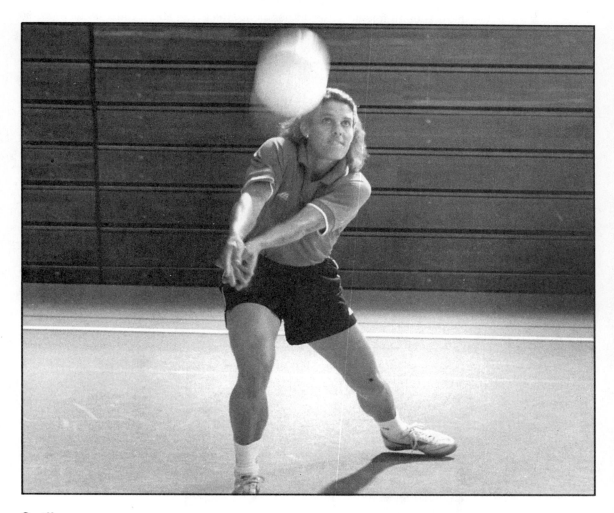

Outline

Defense is as much an attitude as it is a learned skill. Players should obviously achieve good position and skills, but they must also have an attitude that makes them eager to pursue balls that do not go directly to them.

Executing an Effective Defense

The *skill part of defense* is a combination of balance and the ability to rebound the ball up on the player's side of the court with control. The pass must be high enough for the setter to handle it effectively, and it must be targeted so that the setter can play it from the desired area.

Positioning is extremely important prior to the opponent's attack. The defensive positioning on the court is determined by the type of team defense being used. (This subject will be discussed more fully in Chapter 11, Team Defense.)

The *ready position* begins with the feet about shoulder width apart, and the weight forward and on the toes. A slightly staggered stance with the right foot forward is the preferred method because it standardizes the fundamental. If the right foot is always forward on every contact, the player doesn't have to learn the different weight shift that would be necessary if the left foot were sometimes forward.

Some teachers prefer that the outside foot be forward, because it might help the player to pass back into the court. This allows for "on help" (meaning that there is help on the inside of the court if a mistake is made on the pass).

The defensive player may be in a stationary position or may pre-hop just prior to the ball being contacted by the attacker. This is similar to the action of a tennis player preparing to receive a serve. The stationary position is recommended because the pre-hop often takes the weight from the toes and shifts it to the heels (the least desired weight distribution).

**Individual defense
ready position**

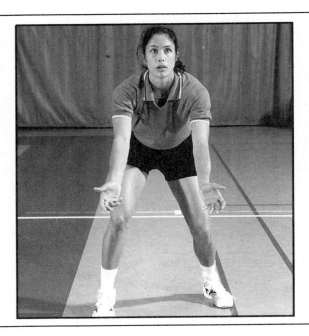

a.

b.

c.

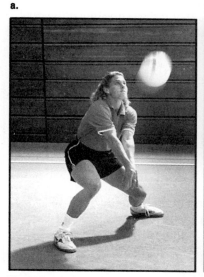
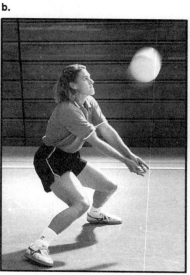
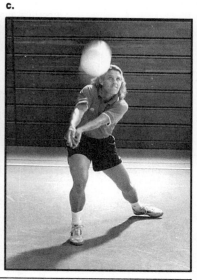

Digging:
a. posture for digging
b. posture for digging
a hard driven spike
c. posture for digging
a ball outside the
midline of the body

The arms extend in front and away from the body. They should be in the passing position prior to the contact of the ball. The keys to digging with control are to keep the rebound angle of the arms always pointing up and to move the feet so that the ball can be played in the midline of the body. This movement to the ball is called the "stride," or "lunge."

This striding movement should be used to get low and under the ball. The foot closest to the ball leads, so the balance and support remains inside the midline of the body. The greater the stride, the better the player's range becomes. The ball should be contacted low and on the forearms. The wrists snap up to

Posture for digging up using the "J" stroke   **Front view of "J" stroke posture**

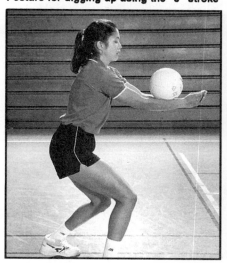
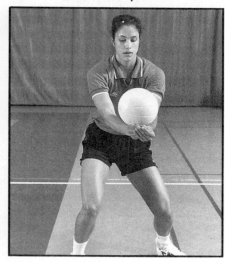

scoop or "J" the ball up with backspin. On harder-hit balls, the player may need to take speed off the ball by cushioning it so that it doesn't rebound back over the net. This action is gained by moving the arms slightly back toward the body upon contact with the ball.

 Checklist for the Save Technique

1. Start in the ready position.
2. Have the outside foot forward.
3. Keep the arms in front of the body and ready to handle the hit.
4. Move the feet so that the ball can be played in the midline of the body.
5. Keep the rebound angle of the arms pointing upward—"dig up, not out."
6. Contact the ball low and snap the wrists up to give the ball backspin.
7. Use an appropriate recovery technique.

The *sprawl* is one of the techniques used to increase the range of one's play. It is used when the ball is outside the range of the player's stride. When executing the sprawl, after extending to the full reach of the stride the player continues to move to the ball by extending the body parallel with the floor. The ball is played outside the midline of the body. The arms are thrust forward and kept parallel to the floor. The ball is scooped just before contacting the floor, and the player finishes the play by laying out flat on the floor.

Striding into the defensive sprawl

Stride and extension prior to contact

Digging the ball with the sprawl

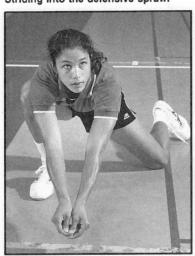 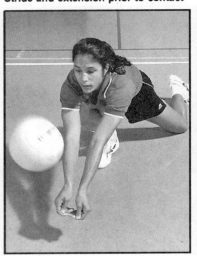 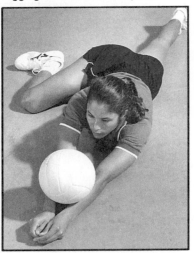

Extending to play the ball

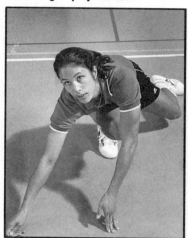

Post contact "log roll"

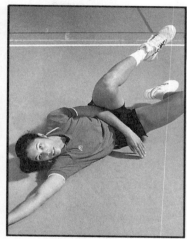

Completion of the "log roll"

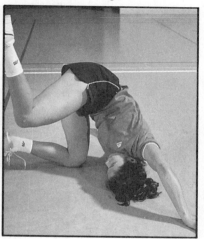

The *dive* is a further extension of the sprawl. In the dive, the player moves toward the ball makes the play and then dives along the floor. This move is used when a player has generated momentum by running after the ball—it is the recovery move used after the ball has been played.

As in all defensive save techniques, the ball should be played as close to the floor as possible. Since the ball is low to the floor, the body will also be low. The play can be made with one hand, but two hands are preferable.

After the ball has been played, the hands are extended to the ground and the weight of the body supported to cushion the landing. As the chest and abdomen get close to the ground, the back is arched and the feet kicked up to avoid dragging the knees and toes. The head is held up to keep the chin from contacting the floor, and the hands are pushed back along the sides of the body to gradually dissipate the momentum of the body weight landing on the floor.

Posture prior to striding to the ball

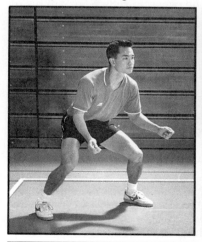

Striding to the ball with second step

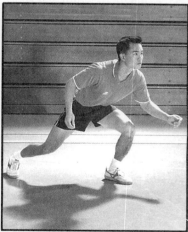

Striding to the ball with second step

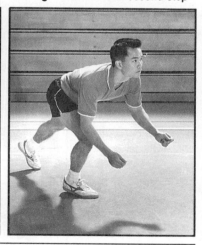

Playing the ball up with a drive

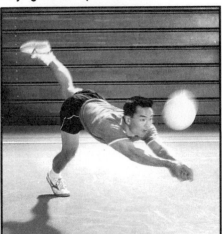

Post dive catch and slide

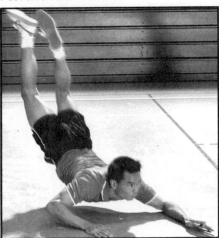

If executed properly, the dive recovery will allow the player to make a good controlled play and then get to the floor with no injury. The recovery should be trained without the ball to ensure proper technique. Once the technique is perfected, the ball can be introduced and the whole process can be practiced.

The *roll* is another save technique. It is used when the ball is beyond the reach of a stride or a sprawl. In the roll the player will once again try to play the ball from the lowest position possible. The stride is made and the body weight extended over the lead leg. The ball is contacted with either one or two hands and the wrist is snapped up to control the ball and give it backspin.

Once the ball has been played, the recovery process is started by the knee of the lead leg turning back toward the body so that the torso is turned to expose the player's back rather than his or her side. From this position there are a couple of ways to continue the recovery: In the log roll, the player simply rolls across the back laterally, and in the somersault roll, the player rolls diagonally across the back and over the opposite shoulder—a back shoulder roll. If performed correctly, this momentum will allow the player to return back to his or her feet.

In any technique the primary consideration is to make the play on the ball first and then make the recovery. Of course, even the best form on the dive or roll is useless unless the ball is properly hit and controlled.

Checklist of Common Errors in Defensive Techniques

1. Moving while the ball is being attacked.
2. Failing to watch the block and the hitter.
3. Not pursuing the ball.
4. Digging the ball back over the net instead of to a setter.

Drills

1. *Two-table multiple contact digging*—Two tables are set up on one side of the net. One person stands on each table and hits balls at the single digger on the other side of the net.
2. *2/3/4 person pass-set-hit*—The teacher or coach stands on a table and hits a ball to a passer who starts the pass-set-hit sequence.
3. *High-set ball defense*—The ball is set high to a hitter. The block forms and the non-blockers set up in their defensive alignment.
4. *Direct-set hitting*—The setter sets the hitter (no pass), and a block forms quickly. Only two contacts are allowed each time.

Checklist for Progression

Beginner:
1. Basic position.
2. Digging the ball up with two arms.

Intermediate:
3. Sprawl.
4. Ball pursuit.

Advanced:
5. Dive.
6. Roll.

Summary

1. Defensive play is as much an attitude as it is a series of skills.
2. The first concern is to position oneself properly, to be able to perform the assigned responsibility for the team.
3. Be in the ready position before the ball is hit by the opponents.
4. Hit the ball as close as possible to the floor.
5. Use the stride, sprawl, dive, or roll techniques to reach the ball and recover from the save.

CHAPTER 10

Team Offense

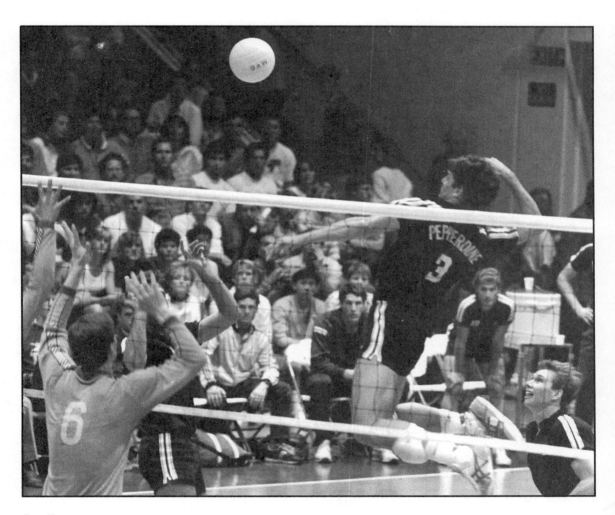

Outline

Overview of Team Offense

Every team will have a basic system with which it works it offense. The system will be determined by the number of hitters and setters employed. Within the system, various formations will be assumed to receive the serve, attack the set ball, and cover the attacked ball.

Serve reception is extremely important because without controlling the serve, the team cannot attack effectively and gain the serve. Team offense begins with the service reception. While receiving service, the rule is that there cannot be an overlap between the adjacent players (refer to Chapter 3). When a serve is hit, the front-row players on the receiving team may not duck under a ball if they are not going to pass it. Instead, the players should "open up" by moving sideways. This will create a passing lane for the back-row passer.

**Court formation
with no illegal
overlaps**

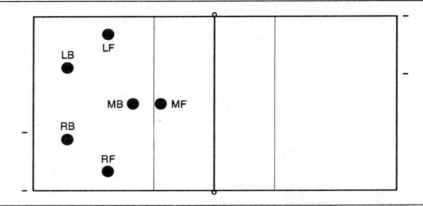

**Court formation
with illegal overlaps**
Middle back must
be behind middle
front.

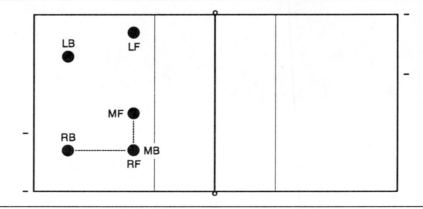

Developing a team offensive system requires that the players' strengths and weaknesses be identified. Once this is done, training should maximize the strengths and hide the weaknesses—hence not every effective team will use the same theory or strategy.

Attack options include getting one or more spikers in a position from which they can successfully attack the ball. At the beginning level, there will generally be just one spiker on each side of the setter. At the intermediate level, a team may employ a single crossing pattern in which a quick hitter and a playset hitter cross, with either of them attacking the ball. (The setter will determine which player receives the set.) At the elite level, there are usually multiple crossing patterns with as many as five possible attackers attacking: three from the front row and two from the back row moving in the pattern at the same time. In this system the setter can predetermine the attack patterns and who will receive the set, or the specialized hitters can call out their attack patterns and the setter can then choose the best option to set.

Split hitters

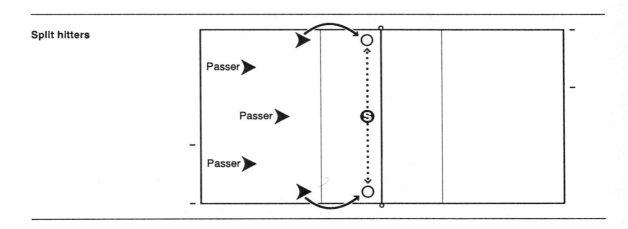

X-crossing pattern

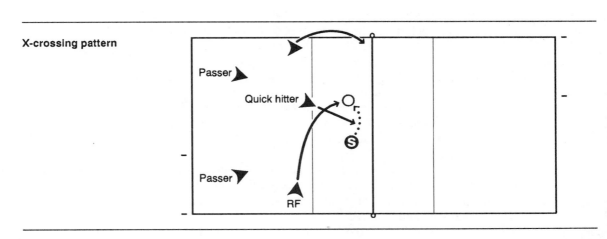

Multiple-crossing patterns

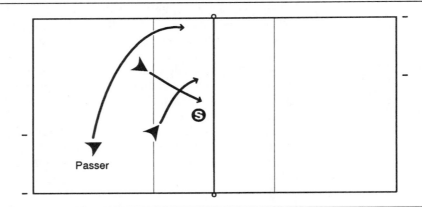

Passer

Advanced patterns

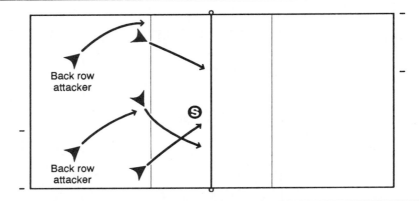

Back row attacker

Back row attacker

Specialization is essential at the higher levels of play. The teacher or coach should determine the strengths of each player and then place them in an offensive scheme that permits those skills to best be utilized. The good passers must be put into positions where they can make most of the passes, the good setter should be doing most of the setting, and, of course, the good hitters should do most of the attacking.

For example, in a 5–1 offense (which will be discussed in more detail later in this chapter) the player opposite the setter could be either a specialized passer or a specialized hitter-blocker who does not set in the normal serve-receive pattern.

As each player practices an area of specialization, he or she becomes far more proficient at that skill. This development technique is a recent innovation in volleyball, but has long been the mode of operation for other sports such as baseball and football.

In developing an offense it is important to *practice in game-related situations*. While drills are important in developing skills, for players at the advanced levels scrimmaging should often be used early in the practice rather than late in the session. The major learning task for the day, whether it be techniques or team play, should also be practiced early when the players' minds are fresh. All too often, team offense is left for the tailend of practice when there is little time or when there is potential for fatigue.

Offensive Systems

Beginner System

The *beginning offensive system* is *6–6 system* of offense. The 6–6 means that all six players may be setters or attackers. Usually the player in the middle of the front court is the setter. After a rotation for the serve, that player becomes the right-side spiker and another player rotates into the middle setting position.

The *serve receiving formation* is the "W" formation. This formation uses three players about 14 to 15 feet from the net, and two deeper players in the seams between them about 21 to 23 feet from the net. The setter aligns near the net closest to the center front (zone 3), being certain not to overlap side to side with the other front-row attackers. The pre-serve ready position will have each passer with the right foot forward, knees slightly bent, and arms in front of the body. By always having the right foot forward only one motor skill is required, no matter which zone is being served.

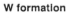

W formation

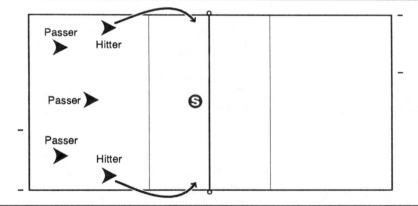

Whatever the serve receiving formation, the players should all be able to see the server and be ready to react to a serve in their respective areas. They should also know who is responsible for calling the lines (when a ball will go out of bounds). This is best done by having the two people deepest in the formation help the others. If the serve is going to the left-back player, the right-back player takes responsibility for making the call.

Both verbal and non-verbal communication among the passers is important, so a player may signal verbally with a call or may make a non-verbal signal by moving to or away from the serve.

In general, the front-row passers should not play a ball that is above waist height; instead, they should let the back-row players take these. Players should also know who will take balls in the seams between them. An easy rule to remember is to have the player on the right of a seam take the balls served into the seam. But individual skills may require a different tactic—perhaps allowing the best passer to handle all balls in his or her area.

Hitter coverage is the action in which the attacking team members align to cover their court in the event that the spiked ball is blocked back into their court. In general, the receiver will pass the ball and then follow it to the net.

Hitter coverage

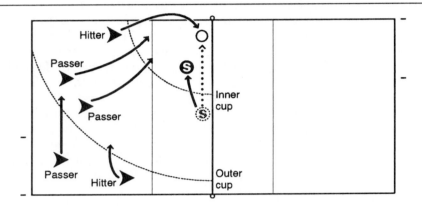

In hitter coverage, the eyes of the players should be on the arms of the blockers instead of the flight of the ball from the spiker to the block. This is because it is much easier to focus on the ball as it comes off the block than as it leaves the hitter's hand before bouncing off the block. In any system of play, the hitter coverage formation should include an inner cup and an outer cup.

In the 6–6 system, the inner cup (three players closest to the attackers forming a semi circle) will include the setter and the two back-court players nearest the attacker. The non-hitting attacker and the deepest back-court player play the outer cup. So if the attack is from the left forecourt (zone 4), the setter, the left back, and the center back form the inner cup and the right-front attacker and right-back player form the outer cup. (Players furthest from the attacker who form a secondary line in the seams between the members of the inner cup.)

The advantage of the 6–6 system is that everyone gets to play every position and it is very simple. It gives beginners a chance to understand the game. The disadvantage at the higher levels of play is that the players generalize rather than specialize, so they are not able to adapt to their best positions. A short player who may have the potential to be a good setter gets to set only once in the six serve-receive rotations.

Intermediate System

The *intermediate system* is the *4–2 system* of offense. With the 4–2 system there are four attackers and two setters. In this system a setter will always be in the front row, so there will be only two attackers in the forecourt positions.

4-2 offense

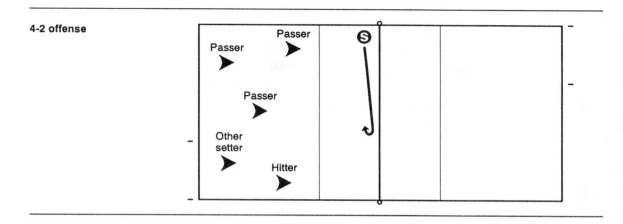

At the lower intermediate level the setter will generally be positioned in the middle of the front court—approximately ten feet from the right sideline. The attackers will be split on either side of the setter. If the setter is in a side zone the attackers will align in the other two zones, to the inside of the setter.

Middle setter

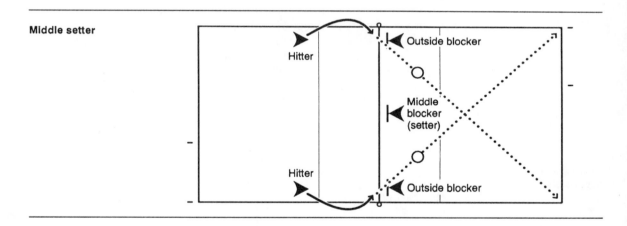

Advantages of the middle setter scheme include:

- The wider spiker has more area on the diagonal in which to hit the ball (42 feet across the court).
- The spiker has a better chance to intentionally hit off the block and out of bounds.

Advantages of side court setter scheme include:

- It puts pressure on the middle blocker to first protect against an attack from the middle spiker and then move to the side if the set goes to the widest attacker.
- An attack from the center of the court is effective against some players.

- For teams who switch players into the block because they don't like their setters being involved in blocks at the center, this alignment of the offense reduces the possibility of such switches.

International 4-2

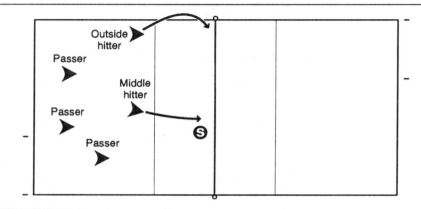

If the setter sets from the right-front zone (zone 2), the spiker who will play the left-side zone (zone 4) for two rotations [because he or she started in the left zone or switched with the setter who started in the center zone (zone 3), then moved to the left zone (zone 4)] is called the "on-hand" hitter. The spiker who stays twice on the right side [starting in the right zone (zone 2) or switching with the setter who started in the right zone] is called the "off-hand" hitter.

The *serve receiving formation* for the 4–2 is commonly the "W" formation. (See the 6-6 formation above.) The 4–2 responsibilities are shown in the following diagram.

4-2 W serve receive responsibilities

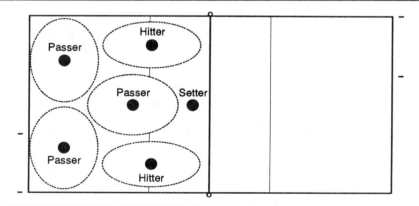

General advantages of the 4–2 offense include:

- There is less movement by the players, so theoretically errors are reduced.
- Less skilled players are more likely to be more efficient.

- It is a simple system, so tactics are usually easy to employ.
- It allows the small player to remain active in the game.
- It requires only two good hitters (because one can always be in the front line).
- The hitter coverage is strong.
- Passer accuracy is not as critical as in other schemes, since there is a larger target area (because the setter is always in the front row).
- It is a good system for an inexperienced coach.
- It is a good system for inexperienced players.

Disadvantages of the 4–2 offense include:

- The difficulty in deceiving opponents with only two major attackers in the front row.
- There are only two attackers versus three blockers.
- Sets are received from two different setters, so the setters and hitters are not as familiar with each other.

In order to reduce these disadvantages good teams will make passes to the setter that are high enough to allow him or her to attack or set the ball. With a setter who can spike, the offense gains another option and the defenders have another element to deal with. This is a prime situation for the setter to use a jump set, because the blockers don't know whether to defend the setter's spike or to defend against the remaining two hitters.

Hitter coverage in the 4–2 offense tends to be consistently strong because there are only two attackers to cover. The shift to the inner and outer cup responsibilities are the same as those explained for the 6–6 system.

When designing a *starting lineup* for this offense, the important consideration in placing the players is balancing their strengths and abilities. In thinking of the six zones on the court, the best attacker will be opposite the second-best attacker. The fourth-best hitter will be one zone clockwise of the best hitter. The third-best hitter will be opposite the fourth-best hitter. The best setter will be one zone clockwise of the fourth-best hitter. The second-best setter will be opposite the best setter. (See the diagram.) The intent is to position the two best hitters so that one will always be in the front row.

**Typical starting
position for a
4-2 offense**

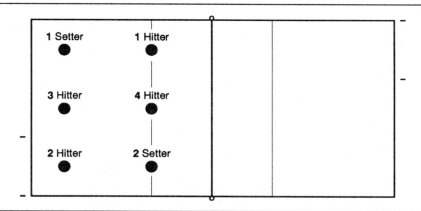

The actual zones that the players will take at the beginning of a game may depend on several factors. The coach may want the strongest server to be the first server, or perhaps it is more important to have the best hitter start in the left-front court. If, for example, the best server is also the best attacker, the coach will have to choose between these two initial starting positions. But in either case the forementioned relationships will remain intact. Another possibility in how the rotation will start might be that the coach wants to receive serve and then rotate into the team's strongest blocking and defensive position.

 Checklist of Common Errors in Team Offense

1. Trying to play with a system beyond the team's skills.
2. Failing to evaluate players' strengths and weaknesses.
3. Not utilizing each players' potential because of the specific system's limitations.
4. Not developing skill specialization for the individual team members.
5. Improperly using players in the starting lineup.

Advanced Systems

Advanced systems of offensive volleyball are the 6–2 and the 5–1. In the 6–2 system, all six players may be attackers but two are designated as setters. Currently at the elite level, a 5–1 is more commonly used; in this system there are five attackers and only one setter.

The *6–2 system* uses a back-row player as the setter so that all three of the front-line players can be attackers. They can be employed in a variety of different alignments and patterns.

6-2 offense
The two setters who are opposite each other come out of the back row to set. The three front row players all hit.

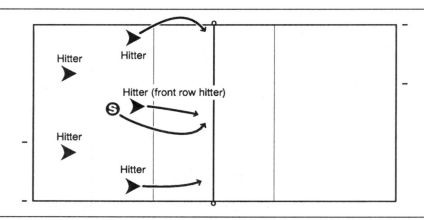

Advantages of the 6–2 offense include:

- There are more front-line attackers (three).
- The three attackers are better able to defeat three blockers.
- With three attackers it is tactically easier to attack the entire length of the net.
- There are multiple offensive possibilities.
- Players frequently prefer a three-hitter attack, and thus will usually work harder to perfect it.

Disadvantages of the 6–2 offense include:

- All six players must be adequate hitters.
- The serve must be received accurately.
- The setter must hit as well as set.
- The hitters must be able to adjust to the sets of two different players.
- Transitions are more difficult for inexperienced teams.
- It takes more time to perfect.
- Because the system is more difficult, players may blame the system for their own poor play.
- This system requires more jumping, more conditioning, and more practice time in order to be effective.

The *serve receiving formation* can be designed to receive with two, three, four, or five players. It is actually easier to receive serves with fewer people, because there is less chance of miscommunication between the potential receivers. The 1984 and 1988 men's Olympic gold medal teams, for example, employed a two-player serve receiving formation. A "W" formation can be employed if five players are to be responsible for the serve reception, four players would play in a semi-circle alignment, and two or three players receiving would be in a straight line (see diagrams).

Hitter coverage for a middle attack would have the setter as the only player in the inner cup. This is because the setter is so close to the middle hitter and the blockers that it is easy for him or her to handle a ball blocked downward. The other four players form a close semi-circle as the outer cup.

Sample 2 man serve receive

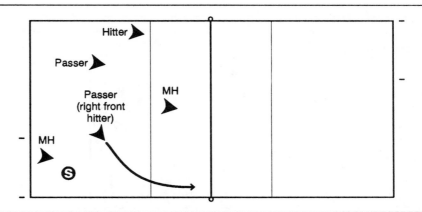

**Hitter coverage
on a quick hit**

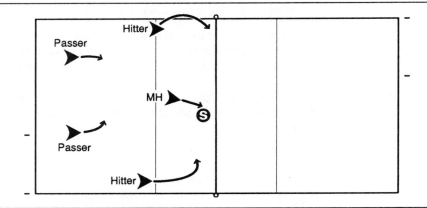

For an attack from the outside if the pass is good and the quick hitter jumps, the setter then moves to the area of the attack and becomes the primary member (the middle position) of the inner cup. The back-row player behind the hitter moves forward and becomes the deepest player in the inner cup. The quick hitter, after landing, moves along the net and becomes the inside member of the inner cup. The closer and lower the set is to the net, the tighter the inner cup will be. The center back and the offside attacker form the outer cup by positioning themselves in the seams of the inner cup but about ten feet behind.

**Hitter coverage for
outside attack with
a quick hitter**

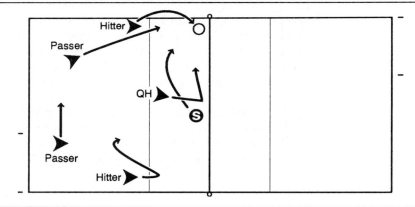

**Right side:
hitter coverage**

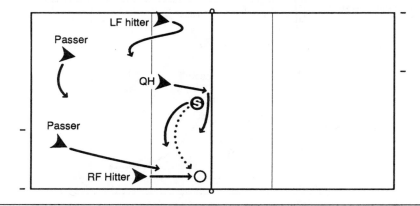

If the pass is poor the setter can't make the quick set, so the quick hitter does not jump. The quick hitter then becomes the primary (middle) member of the inner cup and the setter takes the position by the net. Hence, on a poor pass the quick hitter and setter exchange responsibilities in the inner cup.

Designing a *starting lineup* for a 6–2 offense requires concerns similar to those mentioned for the 4–2. The 6–2 system will generally have two specialized setters, two specialized quick hitters, and two specialized passer-outside hitters. As in the previously mentioned rotation, the setters will be opposite each other. In the rotation the quick hitters will lead the setters and the passer-outside hitters will follow the setters.

Sample 6-2 offense

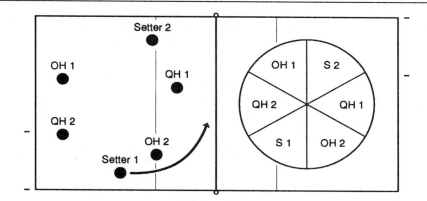

The *5–1 offense* uses one setter and five attackers. It is the most commonly used system in elite-level volleyball, from high school to the Olympics. With the setter in the back court the attack is like a 6–2, with three front-line hitters. When the setter is aligned in the front court it is like a 4–2, with only two primary hitters.

In this system, when the setter is in the front row he or she must be able to jump set as well as tip or hit. With these skills it is hoped that the setter can occupy one blocker.

The setter must be physically, technically, and emotionally fit. He or she must be intelligent enough to understand the complete game and intuitive

5-1 offense

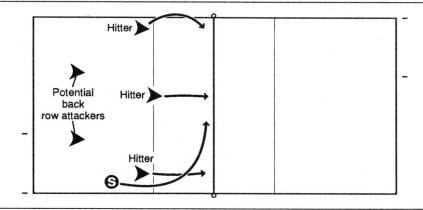

enough to be able to direct the attack in the way most advantageous to the offense. The setter must know who is a "hot" hitter. It is also important to know where the matchups favor the offense so that the hitter chosen will have the best chance of defeating the block.

Advantages of the 5–1 offense include:

- Only one setter need be in control all the time.
- Hitters need only to learn to read (work with) one setter.
- Five hitter/blockers are always in the game.
- There are more potential combinations for attacking.

Disadvantages of the 5–1 offense include:

- A team must have one great setter.
- A team must have an accurate passing game to enable the setter to set, spike, or tip the ball when he or she is in the front row.
- There are three rotations where only two hitters are in the front line.

Formation for serve receiving is the same as in the 4–2 and 6–2 systems. *Hitter coverage* is also the same as in the 4–2 and 6–2 systems, with the exception that all players must be aware of the setter's attempt to attack (tipped or spiked ball on the second contact).

Designing a *starting lineup* for a 5–1 attack allows for more options by the offense than in other systems. The offense can be designed to take advantage of a number of specialized strengths of the team members. For example, the player opposite the setter could be a specialized right-side player, a specialized passer and left-side player, or a quick hitter/back-row attacker.

5-1 offense

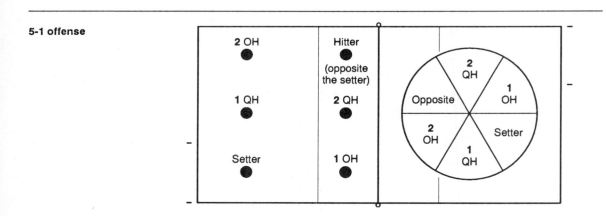

The *swing offense* is a recent innovation in offensive volleyball. It was developed by Doug Beal, the men's gold-medal winning coach for the 1984 Olympics. In the more traditional style of attack, the players move perpendicular to the net when attacking. In the swing offense, the players move laterally and then attack either on the perpendicular or at a diagonal angle. This style of offense makes it very difficult for the blockers to detect who will be attacking and which area will be attacked. Because of this, their movements are delayed and are less effective.

The swing attacker may hide behind the quick hitter and then flare to either side of the court and receive the set. In this offense, the hitters usually call out their attack patterns.

Swing offense

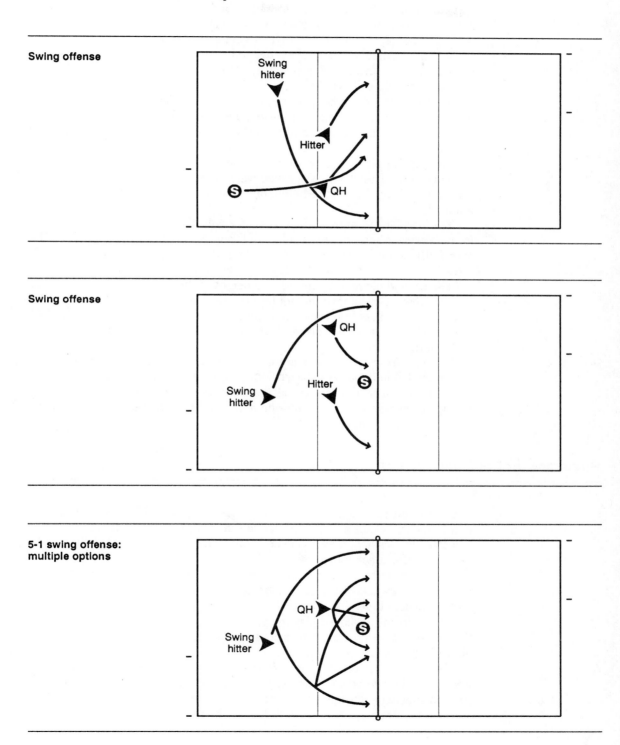

Swing offense

5-1 swing offense: multiple options

Calling Plays

At the beginner level, no play may be called. If one is called, it should be nothing more than telling the player who will attack that the ball is coming that way, such as "Here, Joe" or "Marilyn, it's coming to you."

At the intermediate level, the setter will call the zone of the set from which the ball will be attacked. For example, if the set will be to the left front (zone 4), the call would be "Four."

At the advanced levels, there are many possible elements to a call, such as the area of the net, the height of the set, the path of the attacker, the bunching or spreading of the offense, and the coordination of the front- and back-row attacks.

Calling the plays can be done with hand signals or by verbal signals (audibilizing). The play that is called will tell the area of the net to which the set will travel and the relative height of the set above the net. This is done with numbers.

The standard front-row attack areas for volleyball in the United States call for nine areas along the net. Each area is approximately one meter long. The area farthest left is designated at "1," the next area is "2," and so forth up to area "9." The area is always the first element signaled in a play call.

The second element is the relative height of the set. The second number tells number of feet above the net that the set should reach. So a call of "31" would indicate a set into area 3 that would be one foot above the net. A "95" call would be a set five feet above the top of the net into area 9 (the far right end of the net).

The back-row attack areas are measured along the three-meter line. The line is divided into four equal corridors designated as (from left to right) A, B, C, and D. For a back-row attack all that is necessary to know is the area of the attack, so only the letter is called—no number. The setter and hitter will know the necessary height of the set.

Strategies for Coed Volleyball

Because of the rules differences for coed volleyball, some differences in strategy may also exist. Since a woman player can attack the net or block even if playing a back-court position, a woman who is tall or has great jumping ability can be called into the attack more often.

Generally a man is a better hitter-blocker, so when a man is in the front row he should be switched into the left forecourt as often as possible so that he can be the on-hand hitter.

Just as in any advanced play the setter, who is usually a female, should play the right-back position as often as possible because there is easier access to the net from that point.

Because of the rule that requires that a woman play the ball at least once if it is contacted two or more times, the female players should be positioned as passers or setters. If a male is the designated setter the women must be passers because nearly always the best attacker will be male.

Coed formation

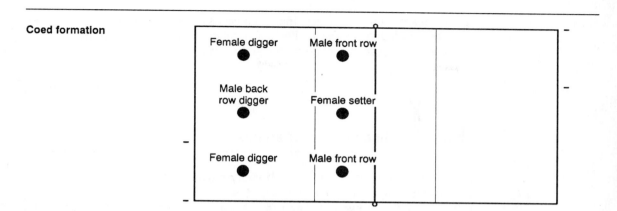

Coed defensive variations

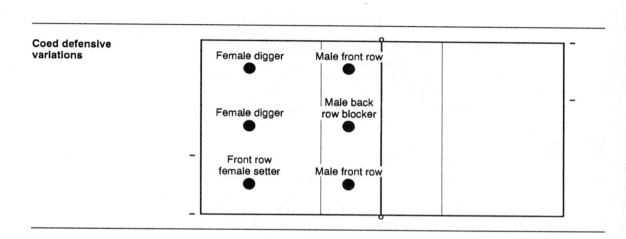

Drills

1. *The rhythm side out*—This is a continuous service-receive drill in which one team continues to serve and the other continues to receive. The teams will rotate on every serve.
2. *Continuous hitter coverage*—This is a drill using a blocking device that will rebound every attacked ball. The attacking team will pass, set, and attack, then play the rebounded ball and repeat the sequence.
3. *Side out with criteria* (Criteria are standards of success such as five total successful plays prior to rotating, or five successful plays in a row.)—The teacher or coach should choose a high level of criteria that is obtainable for the level of the players. After meeting the criteria the team will rotate. The serving team will continue to serve until the teacher or coach calls for a change.
4. *Wash drill*—This is a two-way drill (offense and defense) with each team having an opportunity to score. Team A serves and plays the ball until the rally is over. Team B then serves a ball and plays until the rally is over. If

one team wins both rallies, that team earns a point. If each team wins one rally, it is a tie (a "wash"). The teacher can determine the number of points necessary to rotate or to win this drill.

 Checklist for Offensive Systems

1. The 6–6 is a system in which every player sets and hits, depending on their positions on the court.
2. The 4–2 is a two-hitter attack. There must be four good hitters and two good setters. The set will nearly always come from the setter in the front line.
3. The 6–2 is a three-hitter attack. There will always be three people who can hit in the front line and one setter who comes up from the back line. All six players must be good hitters and two must be good setters.
4. The 5–1 is a combination of the previous two systems. There must be five good hitters and one great setter.

Summary

1. There are several basic offensive systems. They are designated by the number of attackers and the number of setters in the scheme.
2. A 6–6 system is the most common for beginners. In this system each player is a setter or an attacker, depending on their positions on the court during the serve.
3. Intermediate teams may use a 4–2 (four hitters and two setters) system.
4. Advanced teams will use a 6–2 (six attackers, two designated setters) system or a 5–1 (five attackers, one setter) system.
5. Teams must have formations for serve-receiving and hitter coverage.

CHAPTER 11

Team Defense

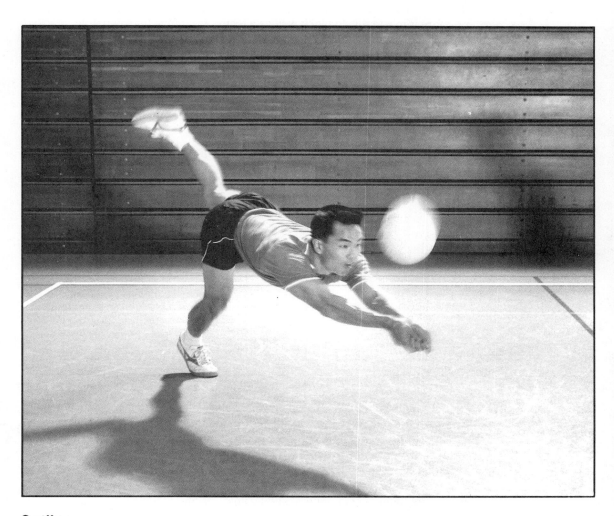

Outline

Introduction

The major job of the defensive team is to score points. All systems and tactics should be based on this premise. Scoring is accomplished by the blockers (the first-line of defense), who terminate attacked balls by penetrating the net and blocking the attack to the floor.

As mentioned in Chapter 8, many teachers and coaches underestimate the importance of training players to technically and tactically block well as individuals or, more importantly, to block well as a team. Continually terminating attacked balls by knocking them to the floor is very intimidating to the unsuccessful attacking team as a whole. Instead, terminating attacked balls or digging and successfully counterattacking the attack team's balls can often change the rhythm of a game or match.

The second line of defense is comprised of the team members not involved in the block. This second line includes the one front-row player not participating in the block, who is called the "off blocker."

Blocking eye contact sequence
1. passed ball,
2. setter, 3. ball set,
4. attacker.

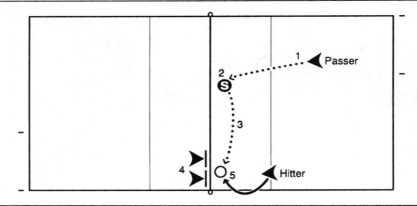

All defenses should be based on what moves the offense is capable of making and what the defenders are capable of executing. A defensive team should not attempt to do tactically what it cannot do technically. Defenses should, as a rule, coordinate the front-row blockers with the second-line players (those teammates not involved in the block). It is the job of the teacher or coach to determine which defensive systems and tactics are appropriate for the team's personnel to employ in general and against specific opponents.

It is common for young volleyball players to be out of balance in their skill development. Usually the elements of offense (the pass, the set, and the attack) are emphasized more than the elements of defensive play. But teachers and coaches should be aware that volleyball is no different from most other sports—the teams with the best defense usually are the most successful teams.

Foundations of Team Defense

Following are some of the foundations of team defense.

Theory:

- Coordinate the second line of defense with the first line.
- Formulate alignments that solidify tip coverage.

Play:

- Players should watch events in this order: the opponent's pass, the setter preparing, the set to its apex, *their own block*, and finally the attacker.
- Dig the ball to the desired target area—preferably to the three-meter line.

Mind set for winning:

- Playing successful team defense (digging, pursuing balls to keep them off the floor, counterattacking) is tough, and success is contagious.
- Teams that are successful should celebrate or at least acknowledge, in good sportsmanship style, their victories.

The *theory and standards of performance* should be developed in the following areas:

Theory:

- Changing the defensive scheme while thinking aggressively makes the offense respond to and worry about your systems, tactics, and personnel.
- Successful counterattacking is essential at the elite levels of volleyball. (The USA men's teams in the 1984 and 1988 Olympics won the gold medals primarily because they were significantly better than the competition in counterattacking.)

Technique:

- The ball should be played with both feet planted, and with two arms on the ball as often as possible.

Mind set for winning:

- High-level teams must develop an aggressive team approach to the defense work ethic.
- A team must adopt an enthusiasm for pursuing all balls that are spiked, deflected, or tipped.
- Communication with teammates must be maintained during play situations such as the standard dig-set-hit sequence and other spontaneous instances.
- "Swinging to score" while counterattacking makes the defensive team more aggressive.
- Adopt the motto: "If we have the ball, the opponent pays."

Defensive Systems

The major job of the defense is to offset or neutralize the spiking attack of the offensive team. This can be done from any of several alignments. While beginners will need to concentrate on playing only one defense, intermediate and advanced players will need more options to stop the more varied attacks of the higher levels of play.

The defensive theory begins with the number of people involved in attempting to block the ball. If the attacking team does not have a chance to spike, no blockers are required. Some situations will require only one blocker, some two, and some three blockers.

Progression of Defenses

The *"W" defense with no blocker* is a defense for beginners who do not know how to spike.

W defense

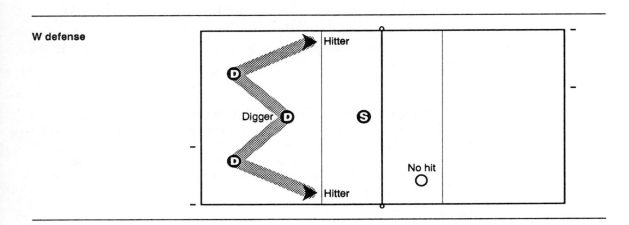

The *"W" defense with one blocker* at the net is a scheme for beginners whose attackers may have the ability to drive the ball down into the defenders' court. One blocker is designated to be at the point of attack and prepared to block the ball if necessary.

1-blocker defense

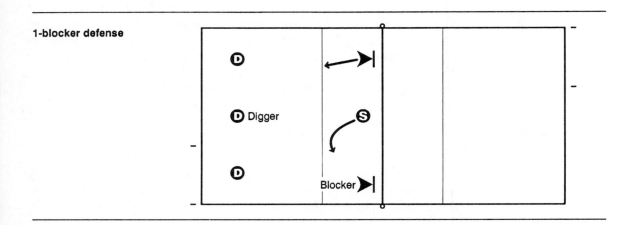

Up defense

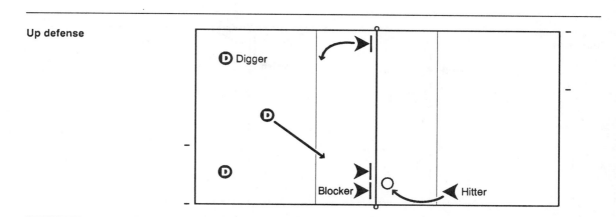

The *up defense* brings a player up from the back row to cover behind the block for any tipped, offspeed, or deflected balls. It is common practice to bring up the center back-row player (zone 6) or the setter, but any back-row player can be the designated "up" player. Some teachers or coaches have their weakest defensive player up because they feel it gets that person out of the way.

The "up" player gets behind the block and straddles the three-meter line. It is obvious from the diagrams that the defensive player in the "up" position does not have to move much and that both the tip and the perimeter are covered.

Most beginning and intermediate teams use an up defense, as do some advanced teams.

The *back* or *perimeter defense* is used primarily against good hitting teams. The weaknesses of this defense are that the middle of the court is vulnerable (in theory, no ball should be hit into this area) and the fact that the line digger on the side of the attacker and the off blocker (the blocker on the opposite side) have dual responsibility for the driven ball and the tipped ball. This dual responsibility often finds these two players moving or charging in as the ball is attacked.

Setter-up defense

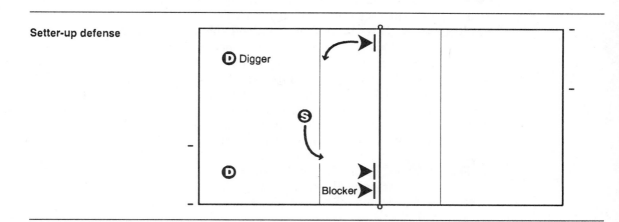

**Back defense:
right side set**

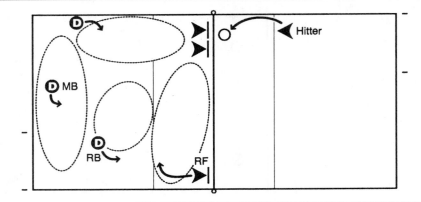

Quick hitter defense

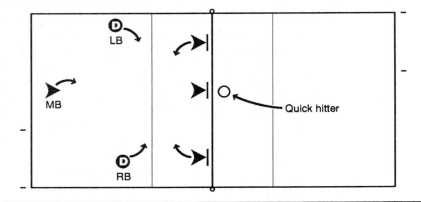

The center back in this defense should not necessarily stay in the exact center back part of the court on every play. Instead, the position of the center back should be based on the abilities of the blockers and the tactics and tendencies of the various attackers.

The off blocker's responsibility is the sharp-angled spike or the tip inside the block. The back-row angle digger usually is positioned to see the ball and the attacker. This player should not be behind the blockers unless it is by design. Often this player is sent to the corner to retrieve deep-corner attacks.

This defense can be used at any level, but requires considerable practice time or experience to cover the offspeed situations that may arise.

The *rotate defense* is a simple but solid defense. The line digger on the side of the court where the attack originates moves up and is responsible for the tip. The center back rotates to the corner vacated by the line digger. The other back-row player moves to the opposite corner. The key player in this defense is the off blocker, who must react to the set and then quickly get to the primary digging position before the attacker contacts the ball.

The two back-row players have flexibility to adjust the court balance for attackers with strong tendencies. Some teams rotate for attacks to one side but not to the other side.

Rotate leftside set

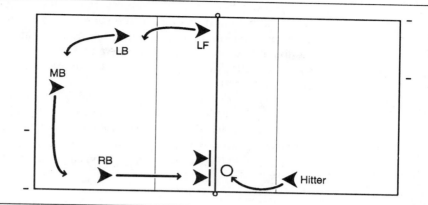

Rotate to right side set

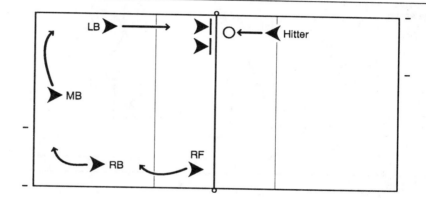

The *slide defense* has the off blocker sliding over behind the block to cover the tip, the offspeed hit, and the deflected ball. The strong point of this defense is that the back-court players have only one responsibility—to play the driven balls. The off blocker (in theory) has all tips.

Slide defense

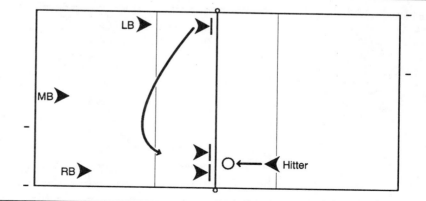

Some teachers, coaches, and players see this defense as hindering a strong counterattacking transition. If the slide blocker happens to be the strongest front-row attacker, that person may not be in position to counterattack. (The argument to this criticism is that the game should be played one play at a time, so counterattacking does not receive a higher priority for the first play than court coverage.)

The *switch defense* is used by some high-level teams as their high set defense. For example, in the case of a high set to the offensive left-front attacker, the left-back defensive player moves over and up to take the tip responsibility. This play can be automatic or audibilized by experienced players. This defense enables the off blocker to be in good position for counterattacking.

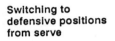
Switching to defensive positions from serve

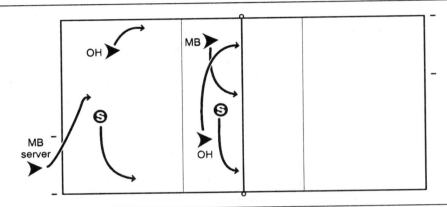

The free ball defense is used when the ball is not spiked and hence a block is not needed. When implementing a free ball defense, the setter moves to the center-front position while the other players resume their service reception formation. The blockers back up, the middle back moves back slightly, and the diggers move farther into the court.

Free ball

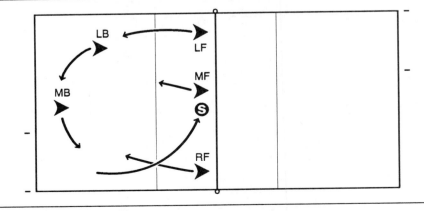

Drills

1. *Positioning*—The teacher stands on a box or a table and hits balls to the areas of defensive responsibilities. Players play out the ball. This can be used with any defense.
2. *Situation defense*—The defensive team has to react to a traditional attack, a free ball, or a down ball shot. The coach or teacher can do this by tossing the ball to an offensive player and commanding that player to perform the maneuver that was called, such as a bump or spike.
3. *The 8 vs. 4*—The teacher or coach continually tosses the ball over the net to the offensive team so that they can run their offensive combinations. The offense needs eight kills to rotate, and the defensive team needs four points to rotate. The scoring can be adjusted to keep this drill in competitive balance. This is an excellent drill because it give the defense numerous opportunities to respond in game-related situations.
4. *Offense vs. defense wash*—See offensive drills in Chapter 10.

Summary

1. The defense must attempt to score.
2. Beginners usually play only one defensive alignment, but more advanced teams will need several types of alignments to be able to stop the various attacks and strengths of their opponents.
3. The common defenses are the "W" with no blocker, the "W" with one blocker, the up, the back, the rotate, the slide, and the switch, and the free ball.

 Checklist for Team Defense

1. The front-row players nearest the attack form the block. (For an attack from the right side of the defense, it would be the right-front and center-front players.)
2. Defensive players should watch, in order: the pass, the setter preparing, the set to its apex, *their own block*, and finally the attacker.
3. All defensive schemes should include the responsibility for tip coverage.

CHAPTER 12

Team Transitions

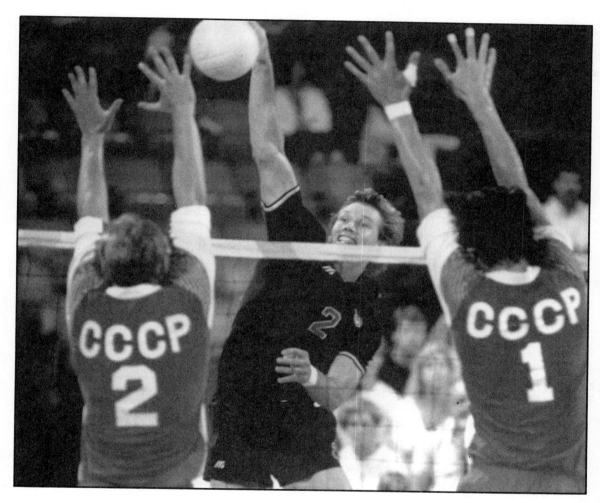

Outline

Service Receiving to Attack and Hitter Coverage
Offense to Defense
Defense to Offense
Checklist for the Individual in Transition
Drills
Summary

Transitions from service receiving to hitter coverage, from offense to defense, and from defense to offense must be done quickly and correctly in order to maximize a team's success. Teams with exceptional talent who don't make effective transitions look disjointed and will not play up to their capabilities, whereas teams with average talent who make good transitions can look like well-oiled machines.

A team should be in either a scoring mode (if it has the serve) or in a side out mode (if it is trying to regain the serve). The difference is that in a scoring mode the team should be more aggressive in order to gain the point, and in a side out mode the play will be more conservative so that the team does not give up a point.

Service Receiving to Attack and Hitter Coverage

When the ball is passed after the serve, the players move forward. As the ball is set, all players "read" the set and immediately react to the set ball. During the set, the non-attacking players move to their positions in the inner cup or the outer cup of the hitter coverage. (See Chapter 10 for a further discussion of offensive moves.)

Offense to Defense

All players immediately react to the attacked ball. The front-row players move immediately to their blocking or spike protection responsibilities. The back-row players move immediately to their defensive responsibilities. They must get back quickly so that their teammates will be in front of them. If they accomplish this, the play will probably be made in front of them. Wherever a player is positioned on the court, it is essential that he or she be stationary, not moving, at the moment that the ball is being hit.

Transition from offense to defense

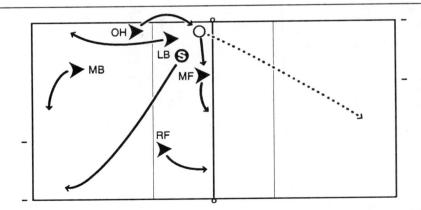

Volleyball is a "forward" game—movements should be made forward. The only reason to move backward is to be in a position to be able to move forward when the moment comes to play the ball. Note, however, that the setter moves back to the designated defensive or blocking position. Many setters will stay close to the net and watch the game instead of switching to defense.

Defense to Offense

All players watch the path of the ball and react accordingly. The transition of the blockers is very important. First, they move quickly to the three-meter line. Once the ball is passed, the back-row players cover the hitter by moving into their coverage positions. This is key—the ball and their teammates must be in front of them. The setter and non-attacking front-row players move into their positions immediately after the set.

Transition from defense to offense

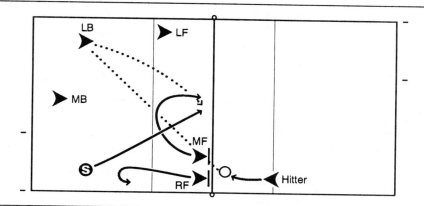

There are three types of transition opportunities when changing from defense to offense: the standard defensive counterattack, the free ball, and the down ball.

The *standard defensive counterattack* is executed when the defense plays an attacked ball effectively, resulting in an opportunity for them to spike. The setter release occurs immediately when the ball is not attacked to the setter's defensive area. In this case, the setter moves to the designated offensive area. If the ball is played to the setter's area, he or she must play it.

Free ball coverage is used when the opponents are not able to attack with a spike. This is generally an advantage for the team taking the offense. The serve reception formation is an effective free ball alignment. The major difference in this instance is that the setter is allowed to play in the preferred setting position and does not have to take a back court responsibility, as might be required in defending a serve.

The setter release occurs when it is certain that the ball will not be attacked. The setter must then move to the designated offensive position. The other defensive players must balance the court when the setter releases.

The *down ball* occurs when the blockers have prepared to block and then decide it is not necessary because the opponents cannot drive the ball down into their court. This can occur when the attacker slips or mistimes the set. The blockers at the point of attack stay adjacent to the net, the off blocker moves to the defensive assignment, and the back-row players move one meter into the court.

The setter release is similar to the standard defense—the setter cannot release until it is certain that the ball will be played by a teammate. The eye-contact sequence of the defenders is to watch the setter, the set, their team's blockers, and then the hitter. It is not necessary to hear the blockers say "down" (meaning that they will stay down on the ground and not attempt to block the ball).

Giving direction in all transition situations is the responsibility of the setter. If the ball is played in a manner in which the setter cannot set the ball, he or she must identify the individual who is to set the ball and the best location in which to make that set. The experienced setter can also give direction to the attackers prior to and during the transition.

The passers are the primary ball control players. They should play as many of the transition balls as possible.

Switching in transition should be done only when there is time to accomplish it. For example, a left-front attacker who has swung to the right to hit may have to remain in that spot for a portion of the rally until there is time to switch back to the left front.

Common errors in making transitions include:

- Not having a mind set geared to scoring.
- Stagnant counterattacks.
- Failure to use the entire net and all attack options.
- Poor communication on the court.

Checklist for the Individual in Transition

1. Know whether you are in a scoring (aggressive) mode or a side out (conservative) mode in your transitions.
2. Watch the ball.
3. React immediately to the position of the ball and to the attack.
4. Be stationary when the ball is attacked.
5. Volleyball is a "forward" game—you move back only to be ready to move forward to play the ball.

Drills

1. *Service receiving to hitter coverage*—This is a continuous hitter coverage drill. See Chapter 10 for a full explanation.
2. *Offense to defense*—Starting with an offensive combination (pass, set, hit), a dug ball is played out. If the spike is killed, the teacher will immediately throw a ball to the defensive team or the offensive team.
3. *Defense to offense*—Start in a defensive alignment with one, two, or three blockers and the remaining players in their correct defensive positions. The teacher or coach gives the offensive team a free ball, tosses a ball for

a down ball situation to the attacker (which cannot be driven down into the opponent's court) or tosses a ball for a traditional attack.

Another defense to offense drill emphasizes repetitive transition. Both the front rows are at the net and the teacher or coach tosses a ball to either side. That side then make the transition from defense to offense.

Summary

1. Making the transition quickly from offense to defense or defense to offense is essential to a team's achieving its maximum efficiency.
2. When switching from defense to offense, the blockers must quickly retreat to the three-meter line and be ready to set, if necessary, in order to counterattack.
3. When switching from offense to defense, the blockers must be alert to the ball and be ready to move toward the opponent's attacker as the set is made.
4. The major transition situations in volleyball are from serve receiving to hitter coverage, from offense to defense, and defense to offense.
5. The transition from defense to offense must take into account whether the team will play a standard defense, a free ball defense, or a down ball defense.

CHAPTER 13

Aerobic Conditioning for Volleyball

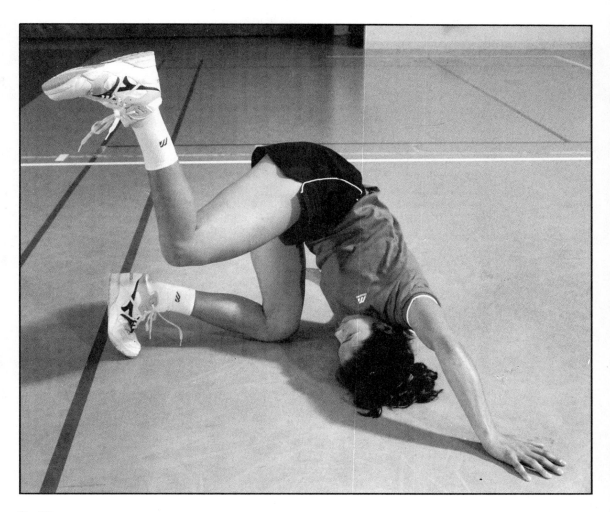

Outline

Proper execution is essential to playing winning volleyball. Fatigue, however, is a prime limiting factor to proper execution.

How many times have you heard the statement, "I blew so many easy spikes," or "I cramped up"? These excuses can often be attributed to fatigue.

Injuries such as pulled muscles (strains), stretched ligaments (sprains), and muscle soreness are often the direct result of fatigue. As players get tired they make more physical errors, thus leading to injury. Being in shape for volleyball can help you avoid these pitfalls and increase your enjoyment from playing the game.

Keys to Getting in Shape

Increasing the capacity of your cardiovascular system (heart, lungs, and arteries) is essential to enable you to supply oxygen to all of your muscles for a period of time long enough to maintain the pace of an extended game or an all-day tournament.

Developing *muscular endurance* is also important. The muscles that are used continually during a match must have the ability to absorb oxygen and other fuels so that they do not tire. The legs (calf and thigh muscles) and the hitting arm (triceps and upper-chest muscles) are most subject to fatigue; therefore they must be exercised for endurance.

Strong muscles are a great help when that extra step, snap, rotation, or support is needed. Specific strength-building exercises can also help prepare the body to withstand the strain of competition with less chance of injury.

Flexibility is also desirable, to enable the execution of quick body twists and all-out reaches without muscle injuries or placing excess strain on joints.

Overload Principle

The main factor in improving fitness of any kind is the *overload principle*. "Overload" means to push yourself each time to do a little more than you are accustomed to doing. Without this factor, there will be no improvement.

There are three ways to overload: intensity, duration, and frequency.

- *Intensity*—How hard you do something.
- *Duration*—How long you do something.
- *Frequency*—How often you do something.

Intensity of exercise may be measured by monitoring your pulse rate, either during or immediately following exercise. The higher the pulse rate, the harder the heart is working. A task should become progressively easier as your condition improves, thus enabling you to work at higher intensities (such as all-out play for a longer period of time).

Intensity means playing at an elevated degree of speed, power, and concentration. All-out play, going full blast for every point, pressing your opponent, and cutting down rest time between serves all put pressure on your opponents.

Duration is measured by how long a period of time you continue to exercise—playing for longer periods of time each time you play, and gradually conditioning the heart to work a little longer each time without rest.

Frequency is measured by how often or how many times a week you play, run, or lift weights. Running four times per week instead of three times is an increase in frequency.

In order to improve the cardiovascular system, you must overload one or more of these principles of fitness. The safest and easiest on the body is frequency. You may overload on frequency by playing more times per week at the same intensity.

Aerobic Training

The cardiovascular system can be improved through the performance of exercises that elevate the pulse rate for an extended period of time. These activities, known as *aerobic exercises*, increase the body's ability to supply oxygen to its cells.

In order to contract muscle cells need fuel, which they receive from blood cells in the form of nutrients. The nutrients are metabolized from the food we eat. Oxygen is necessary in order for the cells to utilize these nutrients. When the heart and lungs cannot supply oxygen at a rate fast enough to keep up with the demands placed on them by the body (a phenomenon known as *oxygen debt*), fatigue sets in and efficiency decreases.

Aerobic exercises train, or condition, the body to adapt to this demand by strengthening the mechanisms involved—the heart, lungs, and arteries. They do this by forcing the heart to work much harder than normal for 20 to 30 minutes.

A *training effect* increases the efficiency of the lungs, allowing them to process more air with less effort; adds to the efficiency of the heart, allowing it to pump more blood with each stroke; multiplies the number and size of the small blood vessels (capillaries); increases total blood volume; and improves the tone of your muscles and blood vessels.

The bottom line is that exercising aerobically increases maximal oxygen consumption by improving the efficiency of supply and delivery. You may select any activity that maintains your pulse in the target pulse zone for an extended period of time. The most commonly recommended activities are running, jogging, cycling, stationary running, rope jumping, walking, and swimming.

Aerobic activities are those that elevate the pulse rate to a level high enough to attain a training effect, but not so high as to cause fatigue or the need for a rest. The individual should be able to continue the exercise for a length of time long enough to attain a training effect.

Target Pulse Rate

One way to ensure that you are exercising aerobically is to monitor your pulse rate to keep it in the *target pulse zone*, the pulse level the body should maintain to reap the benefits of aerobic training. To determine your target pulse zone, first find your maximum exercise pulse, which is determined by subtracting your age from 220. Your target pulse zone is between 65 and 80 percent of your maximum exercise pulse. If the exercise is too intense, your pulse will rise above the upper limit of your target pulse zone and your breathing will become more difficult as a result of your body's attempt to keep up with this extreme oxygen demand. An example is:

$$220$$
$$\underline{-20 \text{ years old}}$$

$$200 \times 80\% \ (.8) = 160$$
$$200 \times 65\% \ (.65) = 130$$

The target pulse zone is between 130 and 160.

This 20-year-old person should maintain a pulse rate of 130 to 160 for 20 to 30 minutes for the body to receive the benefits of aerobic training. This should be done a minimum of three or four times each week.

The key to being able to receive maximum benefits from aerobic activities is to exercise longer, not harder; low-intensity, long-lasting, continuous aerobic training periods help your body become able to continue performing for longer periods of time and to delay the onset of oxygen debt and fatigue while playing volleyball.

Anaerobics

Anaerobic Exercises

Another type of exercise is that which demands oxygen at a faster rate than the body can provide—*anaerobic exercises*. Anaerobic literally means "without oxygen." Anaerobic activities are so intense that they cannot be maintained for a long period of time. Exercises or sports involving stop-and-go activity, such as volleyball, tennis, and soccer, usually require both aerobic and anaerobic conditioning because they have periods of intensity and times of inactivity. They are aerobic because the games last a long time, and they are anaerobic because of their start-and-stop nature.

Examples of anaerobic activities are running a 100-yard dash, weightlifting, or continuous long rallies in volleyball. After engaging a short time in such activities the individual must stop and rest, usually breathing fast and deep to allow the body to replenish its oxygen stores. During anaerobic activities the pulse may be extremely elevated and breathing irregular (panting).

Anaerobic Training

Volleyball often has periods of very intense activity, so the body must also be conditioned for these bursts of all-out play. Such conditioning may be attained through practice, by playing more intensely for longer periods of time, resulting in an overload.

Other activities that may increase the body's ability to maintain a high intensity level are those that bring the pulse rate above the target pulse zone. Examples of this type of activities are running sprints, bicycle sprints, running up long flights of stairs, continuous jumping, and other explosive activities.

Drills

Training is specific. The best way to get into shape for volleyball is to play and practice volleyball. Drills that require continual running and jumping are best

Checklist Comparing Aerobics and Anaerobics

These two types of activities have contrasting characteristics, as shown below:

Characteristics

Aerobics	Anaerobics
Low Intensity	High Intensity
High duration	Low duration
Pulse slightly elevated	Pulse highly elevated
Continuous, uninterrupted workouts	Workouts interrupted by rests
Regular breathing	Irregular breathing; panting
No oxygen debt	Oxygen debt; fatigue
Burns fat and carbohydrates as fuel	Burns carbohydrates as primary fuel

for accomplishing this. A blocking drill with two spikers (one right and one left) forcing the blockers to block on one side of the court, then quickly move to the other side and block, and then return, is one drill that conditions the player anaerobically.

Summary

1. Conditioning can provide the physical means for a player to be able to maintain a high skill level throughout the entire game and avoid errors and injuries that may be attributed to fatigue.
2. Training is specific. In order to get into shape to play volleyball, you must play and practice volleyball.
3. Volleyball demands improvement of the cardiovascular system, strengthening of the muscles, and an increase of the joints' flexibility.
4. For best conditioning results, the overload principle should be the basis of your fitness program.
5. There are three ways to overload: intensity, duration, and frequency.
6. Aerobic training can improve the efficiency of the cardiovascular system.
7. Aerobic training results in the phenomenon known as a *training effect*.
8. Anaerobic exercises are activities of higher intensity and lower duration, while aerobic exercises are activities of lower intensity and higher duration.
9. In order to benefit from the results of aerobic training, the pulse must remain in the target pulse zone all during the activity.
10. Since volleyball is primarily an anaerobic activity, improved fitness may be gained through playing volleyball at a more intense level for longer periods of time and by activities that duplicate these high intensity demands, such as sprinting, jumping, and other explosive activities.

Checklist of Benefits of an Aerobic Training Effect

1. Increased efficiency of the lungs—the lungs can process more air with less effort.
2. Increased efficiency of the heart—the stroke volume of the heart is increased, and the heart can pump more blood with each stroke.
3. Increased number and size of blood vessels—the arteries become stronger and the capillaries increase in number.
4. Increased total blood volume—the body produces more blood cells to meet greater demands.
5. Improved muscle tone—the muscles become fitter and the muscle layer of the arteries becomes stronger.
6. Fat weight changed to lean weight—the lean body mass (percentage of muscle in the body) is increased.
7. Increased maximal oxygen consumption—the efficiency of the supply and delivery of oxygen to the cells is improved.

CHAPTER 14

Strength and Flexibility

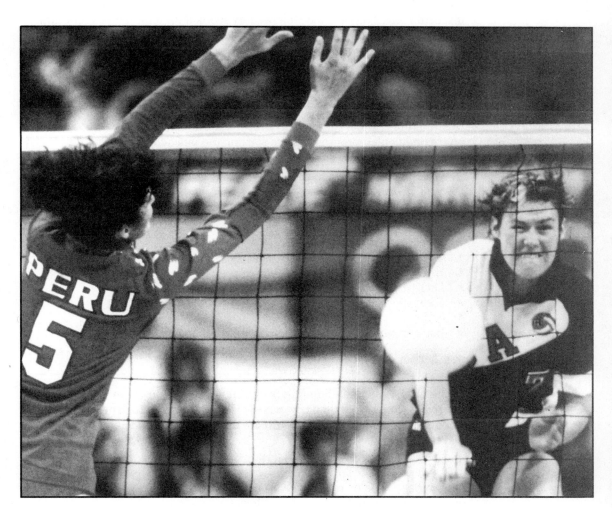

Outline

Volleyball players may not realize how much strength they need for the game. The jumping ability necessary for spiking or blocking a ball or the quickness needed to dig a spike require both strength and flexibility.

Only a few years ago strength training for athletes was taboo; now it is a necessity. The idea that working with weights made people musclebound has given way to the truism that strength and flexibility training are an essential for every athlete.

Male athletes were the first to use resistance training. Shot putters and discus throwers led the way, followed by football players. Soon every athlete, male and female, found that strength training could greatly increase their abilities. As a volleyball player you too can profit from strengthening your body.

The General Strength Program

It should be understood that every athlete should work on a general body-conditioning program before starting the individual exercises.

A general body-conditioning program would include the following exercises:

- Bench pressing.
- Triceps exercises (such as a triceps extension).
- Shoulder (military) pressing.
- Biceps curls.
- Squats
- Calf raises.
- Hip abduction and adduction.
- Lats.
- Cleans.
- Sit-ups.
- Back arches.

The Specific Program for Volleyball

While an overall body-building program may be good for everyone, special exercises can be particularly beneficial to athletes with special interests. Abdominal and lower-back strength are useful in nearly every sport. Volleyball players should strengthen their shoulders, arms, and wrists, as well as their leg muscles.

Under each label of muscle group (such as front of deltoids, rotator cuff, or abdominals), one or more exercises are listed. (If more than one are listed, you need choose only one of the options for your program.)

Upper Shoulders

The shoulders are involved in every lifting, throwing, and hitting activity. Therefore, they are very important in volleyball competition.

Front of deltoids (shoulders)

1. With a dumbbell in each hand and your palms pointed inward, raise the dumbbells as high as possible. This exercise can be done with both arms working at the same time or alternating.

Checklist for General Muscle Strength

1. Shoulder strength (bench press and shoulder press).
2. Arm strength (biceps curls and triceps extensions).
3. Leg strength (squats and calf rises).
4. Hip (abduction and adduction).
5. Upper back (lateral exercises).
6. Lower back (back extensions).
7. Abdominals (curl-ups).
8. General body (cleans).

2. While standing with dumbbells in your hands and at your sides, lift the dumbbells out to the side and directly overhead with the backs of your hands staying on top of them. (If you turn your hands palms up you will be able to lift more weight, because you will be allowing the upper-chest muscles (pecs) to join in the work. You probably don't want this.)

Back of deltoids (shoulders)

3. While lying face down on a bench, or standing and bending forward at a 90° angle at your waist and with your head on a table or against a wall to reduce the pressure on the lower spinal disks, raise the dumbbells sideways from directly below the shoulders to as far up as they will go. Keep your arms straight.

Rotator cuff

The rotator cuff muscles turn the upper arm in the shoulder socket. These very important muscles come into play in most throwing and hitting actions. They are particularly important in throwing a baseball and spiking a volleyball. Because they are quite small, they are often injured. Therefore, they should be exercised for both maximum strength and injury prevention.

4. While lying on your back on a bench, hold a dumbbell and bend your elbow at a 90° angle to your side. Bring the dumbbell to a vertical position, continue the action until the weight is touching your abdomen, and then return to the starting position. This exercise will work two different actions of the rotator cuff muscles.
5. While sitting on the floor with your left side to the lower pulley of a machine, your left elbow next to your hip, and your left hand on the handle, pull the handle across your body by rotating your upper arm and keeping the elbow bent. From the same position, take the handle in your right hand and pull the handle across your body. Next, change to sitting with your right side to the machine and work each exercise. (Note that they pulleys give you better resistance than the dumbbell exercise illustrated in exercise 2.)
6. While standing bent at the waist and with dumbbells in each hand, pull the weights back toward your waist and turn them to the inside.

Abdominals

Most people are aware of how important it is to have abdominal strength. It helps to keep our abdomens tucked in for better posture. In fact, the abdominals—along with the lower back—are the two most important areas for strength in our bodies.

In athletics the abdominals help to stabilize the pelvis, so they are essential in every action that involves the hip joints—running, jumping, swimming, gymnastics, and the hip rotation in a volleyball spike or serve.

 Checklist for Abdominal Exercises

1. Bend your knees so that your hip flexors cannot contract effectively.
2. If your hips leave the bench or incline board, your hip flexors are contracting.
3. Think of yourself as curling up rather than sitting up.

In order to attempt to isolate your abdominals, you should bend your knees as much as possible so that the muscles that flex the hip joint (bringing the thighs forward and upward) will not work as much. You should also keep your hips (your belt) on the mat when doing an abdominal exercise. Whenever your hips are pulled off the mat or bench, your hip flexors are working. This can be particularly harmful for female athletes, who generally have an excessive curvature in their lower backs. [This curvature places a higher pressure on the outside of the disks in the lumbar (lower back) region. It can cause many problems as the person grows older.] The reason that some hip flexion exercises can increase the curvature of the spine is that there are some muscles deep inside the pelvis that attach from the lower-back bones to the thigh bone. As they get stronger, they pull in on the lower spine and increase the curvature. You will often see this extreme lower-back curve (technically called *lordosis*) in female gymnasts.

1. Abdominal curl-ups are done by lying on the floor or on a bench with your knees bent and your hands on your chest. Curl your shoulders forward until your hips are about to leave the floor. Usually you will be able to touch your elbows to your thighs. If you do the curl-ups on an inclined board with your head lower than your feet, you will increase the resistance you are lifting.

    If you are working for strength you should hold weight plates on your chest in order to increase resistance. But most people are looking for muscular endurance so that they can hold their abdominal muscles flat longer. If this is what you want, just do lots of curl-ups (without the weight plates).

    Some people aren't sufficiently strong to do this exercise correctly the first time. If this is true for you, there is another way to do the exercise.

Grab the backs of your thighs with your hands and pull yourself up to the proper position. When you've done this a number of times and it becomes easy, use only one hand on one thigh to help you curl up. Soon you will be able to do the exercise without using your hands to assist you. The exercise is easier with your hands on your hips, and harder with your hands on your chest.

2. Side sit-ups are done to get additional strength in the muscles on the side of your abdominal area (the obliques). For this exercise you will have to have your feet held down. (Someone can hold them for you, or you can hook them under a barbell.) Lift your shoulders from the mat or bench as far as your range of motion allows. This exercise will not only work the abdominal oblique muscles, but also the muscles on the side of your lower back and the rectus abdominis on the side to which you are bending.

Lower Back

Exercises for the lower back are probably the most important for the average person to do, because lower-back injuries, especially muscle pulls, are so common. The problem is that these muscles don't show when we are in our shorts so we often overlook them.

The lower-back muscles are particularly important in volleyball because of the quick bending movements involved. And, of course, they are essential in maintaining good posture, because they are the muscles that hold our chests up by lifting our ribcages. They pull the back of the ribcage down, which raises the front of the ribcage and, thus, our chests.

1. Back arches can be done on the floor. Just stretch out face down and raise your shoulders and knees slightly off the floor. You do not want a big arch, because hyperextending the backbone is not safe.
2. In your gym there may be a Roman chair available. If so, working with this will increase the resistance you can gain in your exercise. In the Roman chair you will put your hips on the small saddle, hook your feet under a bar, bend forward at the waist about 30° and then straighten your back, being careful not to hyperextend.

    If you desire strength, just hold weight plates or a dumbbell behind your head. If you want muscular endurance, just do as many repetitions as you can.

Hip Flexors

The hip flexors bring our thighs forward, so they are essential in any running or jumping activity. As previously mentioned, hip flexion exercises might be harmful for some people, especially females. However, many people need strength in the hip flexor muscles—volleyball players, like anyone who runs fast, must have hip flexor strength.

For those who would be susceptible to an excessive lower-back curvature, special precautions should be taken. Such people should keep the connective tissue in their lower backs flexible by doing toe-touching exercises while sitting. They should also keep their abdominals strong to reduce the tendency of the front of the hips to drop forward. (This tendency would increase the curve of the lower spine.)

Hip flexors are exercised when the thigh is brought forward. This can be done several ways: you can do them hanging or standing, without weights, with a weighted boot, or with an ankle attachment from a pulley on a weight machine.

1. While hanging from a high bar with both hands, bring your legs forward with your knees bent. Touch your knees to your chest.
2. While hanging from the high bar with both hands, bring your legs forward without bending your knees.
3. Using the lower pulley of a weight machine, hook your ankle into a handle or use an ankle strap to secure your ankle to the pulley. Then raise your leg straight forward.
4. While standing (with or without weight boots), brace yourself with your arms and lift one leg forward as high as it will go. Bring it up slowly.
5. Leg lifts are done from the supine position (on your back). Lift one or both legs from the floor to the vertical position. Your abdominals will contract isometrically in this exercise, as in all other hip flexion exercises. Be certain that your back does not arch.

Wrist Flexion (Front of Forearms)

The wrist flexors are used in any throwing or hitting motion. They put the curve on a curve ball and the speed in a fast ball, and they bring the hand through the ball on a spike or serve. Wrist strength is also essential for setting the ball.

1. Sit down while straddling a bench. With a barbell in your hands, your palms up, and the back of your forearms on the bench, let the weight of the barbell hyperextend your wrist, and then flex your wrist forward. This exercise can also be done with a dumbbell, exercising first one wrist and then the other.

    Some people will perform this exercise using a weight attached by a rope to a handle. The exerciser raises the weight by rolling the handle using alternate wrist movements. This is not good for maximum strength gain, but it is all right for increasing muscle size or muscular endurance.
2. An exercise that will assist you in developing wrist strength and also develop strength in your fingers is the tennis ball squeeze. Find an old soft tennis ball and squeeze it repetitively, as fast and as long as possible until fatigue sets in.

Wrist Extension (Back of Forearms)

The wrist extensors are important in stabilizing the wrist in any sport requiring backhand action, such as tennis, racquetball, or golf. In volleyball they hold the hands back while a player is making the passing platform. They are also essential in weight lifting, because they tend to be the weakest link in the "cleaning" action that brings the bar from the floor to the chest.

While sitting and straddling a bench (as in the foregoing exercise) and with your hands grasping the barbell (palms down), let the barbell flex your wrists and then extend your wrists upward. This exercise will strengthen the back of your forearms. You will probably be able to use only about $2/3$ of the weight you were able to handle in the first wrist flexion exercise.

Hip Abduction

Hip abduction means moving your leg sideways in a lateral plane. It uses the muscles on the outside of the hips. It is practiced by anyone who wants to move laterally while facing ahead. It is important in volleyball, which is a game involving lateral movement to get into position to hit a shot.

1. If you have an abduction-adduction machine just sit in the seat, hook your legs into the stirrups, and push both legs outward.
2. With a partner, recline on your back with your partner holding the outsides of your feet or lower legs. Push your legs apart as far as they will go as your partner resists.
3. While standing sideways to a pulley machine at the lower pulley station, hook your foot into the handle (or use an ankle strap) and pull your leg away from the machine.

Hip Adduction

Hip adduction exercises strengthen the muscles on the inside of the leg (the groin area). These muscles are also used when moving laterally.

1. With an abduction-adduction machine, sit in the seat, put your feet in the stirrups with your legs apart, and squeeze your legs together.
2. With a partner, start with your legs spread and have your partner put his or her hands on the inside of your feet or lower legs and give you resistance as you squeeze your legs together.
3. On a machine with a low pulley, stand away from the machine and sideways to it. Put your foot in the handle and squeeze your leg in toward your body, pulling the handle away from the machine.

Flexibility Exercises

Flexibility is generally defined as the range of motion of a joint. Every volleyball player, just as every other athlete, needs a certain amount of flexibility. Stretching exercises to gain flexibility can be done very slowly by holding the stretch (static stretch) or while moving (ballistic or dynamic stretch), but should never be done with jerky movements. It is generally recommended that the slow static stretch be used for most stretching workouts.[1]

Flexibility Warm-Up

A few simple flexibility exercises should be done before every weight workout, practice, or game. Such exercises will stretch your connective tissues and your muscles, so that they will be more ready to react efficiently and less likely to be injured during the more intense exercise. Following is the preferred order for stretching exercises:

---

[1]Coaches Roundtable, "Prevention of Athletic Injuries through Strength Training and Conditioning," *National Strength and Conditioning Association Journal* vol. 5, no. 2, pp. 14–19; Coaches Aroundtable, "Flexibility," *National Strength and Conditioning Association Journal* vol. 6, no. 4, pp. 10–22; and S. P. Sady et al, "Flexibility Training: Ballistic, Static, or Proprioceptive Neuromuscular Facilitation?" *Archives of Physical Medicine Rehabilitation* 63, pp. 261–263.

1. *Shoulder rotation*—Stand erect with your arms extended out to your sides. Rotate them forward in circles, with your hands making circles 12 to 15 inches wide. Do this for 15 seconds, then rotate the arms backwards for 15 seconds.
2. *Seated shoulder and chest stretch*—Sit with your legs together, with the back of your legs flat on the floor and your body erect. "Walk" your hands backward to a comfortable stretch position. Concentrate on keeping your upper body straight and emphasize stretching the tissue in the front of your shoulder. Hold this position for 30 seconds.
3. *Groin*—While seated on the floor, put the soles of your feet together and with your hands pull them toward your hips. With your back straight, try to press your knees to the floor. Do this for 30 seconds.
4. *Lower back and hamstrings*—While sitting on the floor, spread your legs outward as far as possible. Keep your back and legs straight with your toes pointed up, and reach your hands as far as possible toward your right ankle. Do this for 30 seconds, and then touch your left ankle for 30 seconds.
5. *Gluteal stretch*—Sit on the floor with your legs together and the back of your legs touching the floor. Grab your right heel with your left hand, pass your right arm under your right calf, and lift your right foot toward the midsection of your body. Keeping your left leg extended and your upper body erect, do the exercise for 30 seconds. Then do the same exercise with your left leg.
6. *Rock and roll*—While lying on your back, pull your knees tight to your chest and rock back and forth. Continue for 30 seconds. This stretches your back.
7. *Trunk twist*—While sitting on the ground with your legs straight, bend your right leg, cross it over your left leg, and put your right foot flat on the ground. Reach your left arm around your bent leg as if you were trying to touch your hip. Place your right arm behind you as you slowly twist your head and neck until you are looking over your right shoulder. Hold for 30 seconds, and then do the exercise to the other side.
8. *Thigh and groin stretch*—From a standing position, step forward with your left leg. Lean forward over your left leg while keeping your left foot flat on the floor. Push down with your right leg until you feel a good stretch in your thigh and groin area. You can put your hands on the ground for balance. Stretch for 30 seconds, and then repeat with the other leg.
9. *Triceps stretch*—While standing, pull your right elbow behind your head until you feel the stretch. Hold for 30 seconds, and repeat with the other arm.
10. *Triceps stretch*—With your left hand, pull your right elbow across your chest. Hold for 30 seconds, and repeat with the other arm.
11. *Calf stretch*—Stand three to four feet from a wall. With your hands on the wall, lean into the wall while keeping your legs straight. You should feel the stretch in the back of the ankles and the lower legs. This stretch can also be done without a wall by striding forward, bending the forward leg and keeping the rear leg straight.

Checklist for Workout Progression

1. Do a general body warm-up, such as jogging, running in place while swinging your arms, or jumping jacks.
2. Do the stretches specified in this chapter.
3. Practice your movements (such as a serve or spike) slowly at first, so that your muscles warm up effectively.

Summary

1. Every athlete should perform a general body strength workout, which includes exercises for the shoulder, biceps, triceps, abdominals, upper back, lower back, hips, and legs.
2. Every athlete should develop the specific strength, flexibility, muscular endurance, and cardiovascular endurance necessary for his or her chosen sport.
3. All volleyball players should exercise the specific muscular actions that are specially designed to improve success in this sport.
4. The abdominal and lower-back areas are extremely important for strength.
5. Volleyball requires that the player who wants to achieve the maximum potential should do specific exercises.
6. Stretching is needed to allow a person to be able to move in a full range of motion.
7. Stretching is an essential part of any warm-up.
8. Stretches should be held at least 15 seconds, and are even more effective if held 30 seconds.
9. Stretches should be done slowly and held at the maximum stretching position (static stretch).

CHAPTER 15

The Mental Side of Becoming a Better Player

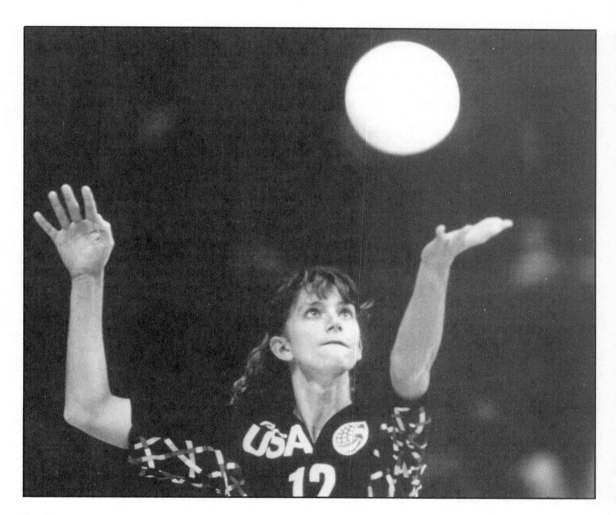

Outline

Mental Practice
Checklist for Learning to Relax
Checklist for Concentration
Checklist for Mental Imagery
Goal Setting
Summary

Wishing won't make you a better volleyball player—you must learn and practice the physical skills of the game. This practice will take place primarily on the court. While it is important to work out physically to condition your body, you can also become a better player at home, by practicing mentally. There are many skills to learn in volleyball and there are so many ways to practice that you should always be able to help your game in some way.

Mental Practice

Championship athletes have known for years that mental practice can help performance. Only recently have sports psychologists refined methods of utilizing the mind's contribution to the game. *Mental imagery*, or *visualization*, are the names given to this type of mental practice. It can be done externally—observing volleyball players or a videotape, or imagining watching yourself from outside your body. (Golfer Jack Nicklaus calls this "going to the movies.") It can also be done internally—"feeling" yourself doing the action.

While mentally experiencing your game, you can practice your sets and spikes, your footwork, or even strategy and court positioning. You can practice whatever aspect of your game you would like to improve. If your service return is a problem, imagine yourself ready for it. The imaginary opponent tosses the ball and serves to your left. Feel yourself making the proper play. Move toward the ball, get your arms in proper position, watch the ball, and make the perfect pass. Think of keeping your head down and eyes focused on the ball.

The following study serves to illustrate how mental imagery can help your game.[1] Basketball players were divided into two groups. The first group physically practices 100 free throws per day, while the second group was placed in a dark, quiet room and told to imagine that they were successfully making 100 free throws. When the two groups were tested at the end of the study, the second group shot for a better percentage. Analysts believe this resulted from the second group's mental imagery, in which they were successful in 100 percent of their shots, while the other group that was actually shooting missed some of their throws, and therefore were not as confident when it came to the actual test.

When using this technique in volleyball, imagine yourself doing everything correctly from start to finish, being sure to include a successful outcome. Perform the action at full speed in your mind, and use as many senses as you can. For example, if you were going to play before a large crowd you might play crowd noise on a tape player in the background as you mentally practiced your skills before the match.

Relaxation is another essential facet of good volleyball. Practice taking a slow, deep breath before preparing to serve. This can help clear your mind so you can concentrate on the serve, and can also help to relax your muscles between periods of action. Relaxed muscles are more prepared for the quick movements essential to playing the game of volleyball. (Tense muscles tend to inhibit smooth, efficient activities and speed up the onset of fatigue.)

To teach yourself to get the most out of relaxation and deep breathing, sit quietly in a chair with your eyes closed and concentrate on slowly taking and

---

[1]Daniel Elon Smith, "Evaluation of an Imagery Training Program with Intercollegiate Basketball Players," unpublished doctoral dissertation, University of Illinois at Champaign–Urbana, 1986, pp. 91–104.

Checklist for Learning to Relax

1. Sit completely relaxed in a comfortable chair in a quiet room.
2. Close your eyes.
3. Slowly take in and release a deep breath while repeating a meaningless syllable.
4. The meaningless syllable repetition should help you to relax by blocking all tension-causing thoughts from your mind.
5. Don't worry if other thoughts come into your mind—just get back into your breathing pattern and your repetition of nonsense syllables.

releasing deep breaths. You can say to yourself "breathe in, breathe out" or repeat a nonsense syllable such as "om" or "one." Concentrating on this syllable repetition is designed to help you relax by eliminating all tension-causing thoughts from your mind. By "not thinking" as you concentrate on your breathing, your muscles will relax and your blood pressure can be lowered. If other thoughts come into your mind, return to your breathing pattern and verbal repetition. This is similar to the Hindu practice of meditation, and is the basis for many of the benefits one can gain from that practice.

After you have learned to relax while sitting calmly in a quiet place, the next step is to transfer that ability to volleyball practice, both on and off the court. You should be relaxed whenever you practice mental imagery, and you should also be able to relax on the court. A relaxed body is more ready to react than a tense body.

Since deep breathing and "not thinking" are important to total relaxation, you can breath deeply when you are tense during a match. Breathing deeply before serving or between rallies will help you to relax. If there is time and you have perfected the relaxation response, you can take a few seconds to close your eyes, repeat a meaningless syllable, and breathe deeply. This will give you a quick mental and physical rest.

Concentration is the third major area of mental practice. You must have a specific focus in order to play at your maximum potential. That point of focus will vary during a rally.

Generally, the most important area on the court to concentrate on is the ball. Failure to focus on the ball all the way to the point of contact and while it is on your hand or arm is probably the most common and critical error at every level of volleyball. Slow-motion studies reveal that most people take their eyes off of the ball when it is still four to six feet away from them. They look at where they want to hit the ball instead of concentrating on the point of contact of the ball and the body.

As was noted earlier in the text it is sometimes necessary to switch your focus of concentration, such as when blocking—from pass, to setter, to spiker. You must know where to focus in each situation—on the ball or on a segment of a player.

When concentrating on something always keep it positive, such as "Watch the ball" or "I am relaxed." Negative thinking is counterproductive and can cause stress. The player who is thinking "I better not miss another serve" is setting him- or herself up for missing the next serve.

Checklist for Concentration

1. Know what or who should be your focus of concentration.
2. If your focus is the ball, focus on it from the first possible moment until after the ball has left your body.
3. If your focus is to change, such as from pass to setter's arm action to spiker, know the sequence and practice shifting your focus.

Checklist for Mental Imagery

1. Watch top-level volleyball players or videotapes of volleyball skills.
2. Be the star in your own movie, by closing your eyes and performing skills to perfection in your mind.
3. Always see yourself completing all aspects of the skill perfectly, including a successful finish.
4. Practice all aspects of the game mentally as well as physically.
5. Always be positive in your instructions to yourself.

Goal Setting

Another important aspect of the mental side of the sport is *setting both long-term and short-term goals.* Short-term goals assist in achieving long-term goals.

After you decide on your long-term goals, make plans to achieve them. An example of a long-term goal is a desire to be the champion of the semester-end class tournament.

Short-term goals are more measurable. They usually involve improving the specific skill that will enable you to achieve your long-term goal. Examples of short-term goals are improving your floater serve to the back corner or learning to time your jump for the spike.

Once you've set a goal, develop a practice schedule designed to increase your chances of attaining that goal. For example, if you want to increase in your ability to spike the ball in addition to the on-the-court repetition of the shot, you can also include mental practice. Visualize different sets, some low, some high, some making you move from your desired position.

With visual practice you can start your physical practice. Have a partner set you some balls. Analyze what you have done right and wrong on your practice spikes. Then replace the negative with the positive in your mental practice.

Summary

1. The complete volleyball player must make maximum use of his or her mental potentials. There are various off-the-court ways to improve one's volleyball.
2. Mental preparation includes:
    - *Imagery*—A person visualizes the techniques and game situations that may be encountered.
    - *Relaxation*—Helps a player avoid tension and perform to a higher level.
    - *Concentration*—Aids the player in focusing on the ball all the way to the point of contact.
3. Goal setting is important for all areas of our lives. Effectively implemented when planning for improvement in volleyball, it can speed up one's improvement in skills and enjoyment of the game.

Outdoor Volleyball

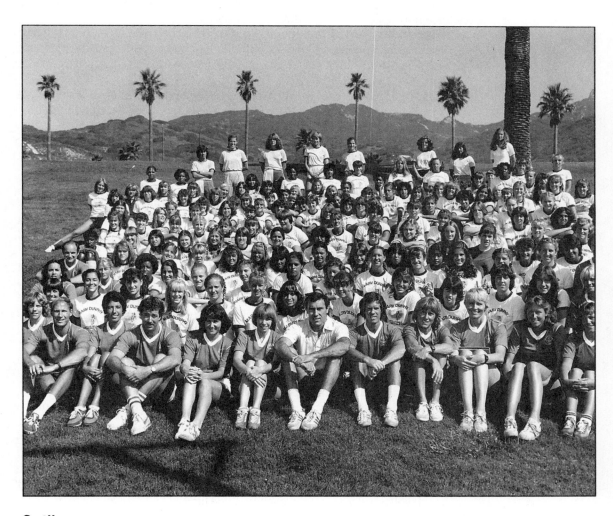

Outline

The United States Volleyball Association sanctions many levels of volleyball play in the United States, from the Olympic team to junior-level play and from high school and YMCA to the professional ranks. Other associations sanction other levels of the game. While different levels of play may have different rules (such as international, women's college, or high school federations), they all are sanctioned by the umbrella organization of the United States Volleyball Association.

Coed play is increasing in popularity as is reverse coed where only the female may spike inside the three meter line!

Professional play is rapidly growing in both the two-player beach game (either men or women) and the six-player indoor game (both men and women). Sports television has increased the interest for the fans and the prizes for the players.

Youth and junior play is the fastest-growing and largest area of volleyball today. There are divisions for players up to 13, for those 14 and 15, and for those 16 and 17.

Whatever the forum, volleyball is one of the hottest sports around.

Outdoor Volleyball

Outdoor volleyball is a common recreational game. Whether it is played at a company picnic or in a professional beach tournament, it is enjoyable and exciting.

Beach volleyball has been played since at least the 1940s. It is played with two people on each team (teams are not limited by sex—they can be made up of two men, two women, or one of each). Because it is played on the sand, the players can dive without fear of being hurt, and because they play the same 30 by 60 foot court dimensions as indoor players, they must be in good physical condition.

The Professional Beach Volleyball Tour, with its newspaper and television coverage, has created both nationwide and worldwide attention. An international professional beach tour has been formed and will soon be operational. Additionally, there is a chance that doubles volleyball in the sand will soon be considered as an Olympic sport.

Playing beach volleyball is not limited to courts along the oceans and lakes of the country—for example, tournaments such as those in Denver, Vail, and Aspen, Colorado, have used sand courts for over 25 years. Many colleges have also built sand courts. Hence the beach has come to the midlands. The sport of beach volleyball was just too exciting to be limited to ocean and lake beaches.

The outdoor ball is heavier than the indoor ball by a few ounces. It is an 18-panel ball, as opposed to the 12-panel ball used indoors. The 18-panel ball is heavier, and as it is usually inflated with less air pressure the wind does not have as much effect on it as it would on the indoor ball.

Some of the *rules differences* for outdoor volleyball are major, and they include:

- Two people per team with no substitutes allowed.
- A match is a single game of 15 points. (Note, however, that this can be changed by a tournament director. 11-point games may be played.)

- Players will switch sides every five points (for example, at a three to two or four to one score) in a 15-point game and every four points in an 11-point game.
- The ball may be served from anywhere behind the end line and between the sidelines extended.
- No open-hand tips are permitted.
- Outdoor players are allowed to stay in contact with a set longer than indoor players without being called for a "lift." But outdoor officiating does not allow for a set ball to spin—that is called a "double hit."
- The ball may be contacted with any part of the body.
- Either a blocked ball or a hard-driven ball can be contacted multiple times in succession during one attempt to play it.
- A player may pass under the net as long as an opponent is not impeded.
- A player may block any ball crossing over the net, including a serve.
- When a player intentionally hits a two-hand overhead pass into the opponent's court, that player's shoulders should be squared up to the ball's line of flight.

Some minor differences include:

- The court is measured in feet (30 by 60), rather than in meters.
- The net height is eight feet for men and seven and one-third feet for women.
- The serve must pass over the net between the poles, versus the indoor game which has antennae.
- The teammate of the server must be within the court and motionless during the serve.
- The server's partner must grant the opposition a clear view of the ball during the serve and, if asked to move to open a visual path, must comply.
- Each player will serve continuously until there is a side out. On the next service opportunity the partner will serve.
- If a player serves out of order, he or she is allowed to continue serving for the duration of that service. There is no penalty for serving out of order; however, the partner will serve the next series after the side out.

Grass volleyball uses the same rules for doubles as beach volleyball. When a team has six players, the indoor rules are used.

Considerations for Outdoor Volleyball

In *doubles*, hand signals are used to designate the area of the court the block is expected to take. If playing in the sand, note that the sand reduces the height to which a spiker can jump so the set must be closer to the net. (This makes it easier to block.) The blocker's partner must know where the spiker is likely to hit the ball, and then cover that area.

In the *three-player* game, anyone can spike or block. One player usually blocks while the other two are diggers.

With *four players*, the server is a back-row player and so is not allowed to spike or block. Usually only one player is designated as the primary setter.

With *five players* three are usually designated as front court players and two as back court players.

A *team with six players* uses regular international rules, but often the digging rules are relaxed a bit and the ball is allowed to stay in contact an instant longer than would be permissible in the indoor game.

The Effects of Nature on Outdoor Play

The *sun* becomes a major factor when playing defense or receiving the serve. The high serve (sky ball) or high attacking shot, which force the opponents to look into the sun to play the ball, can be very effective.

The *wind* is such an important factor that a team may choose "side" rather than "serve" in order to obtain the side of the court that faces the incoming wind. The wind blowing into the server will help to force the served ball down and keep it in the court. This is particularly true with a top-spin serve, which will be forced rapidly downward by the wind. The floater serve into a moderate wind will also be more likely to hold the ball up and then let it drop nearly straight down.

The wind can be a disadvantage to the team hitting with the wind. A floater serve will often carry outside the court. In fact, any deep shot may well be carried out of bounds.

A crosswind can aid a spin serve if the player can spin the ball into the wind. For example, a right-handed server with a counterclockwise rotation (server follows through to the right of the ball) will curve the ball left. A wind blowing to the left will accentuate the spin and may give it a curved trajectory two or three times greater than the spin would have imparted on a calm day. Similarly, a right hander following through to the left of the ball, giving the ball a clockwise movement, will gain additional curvature if the wind is blowing from left to right.

Any wind will also have a profound effect on every pass and set. For this reason, the ball should be played lower to reduce this variable.

 Checklist for Doubles Rules Differences for Outdoor Volleyball

1. Players switch sides every five points in a 15-point game.
2. No open-handed tips are allowed.
3. If passing the ball over the net, the player must face the direction of the hit.
4. A player may pass under the net as long as there is no interference with the opponents and their movements.
5. The serve can be from anywhere behind the end line.
6. The ball can be played with any part of the body.

Recreational Volleyball

The *YMCA* has been involved in volleyball since its inception, because the game was invented at a YMCA. Nearly every YMCA and YWCA has a volleyball program. They also hold their own national championships.

Corporate leagues are an expanding area of volleyball interest. Some companies have their own courts; others rent or schedule time on courts at schools or public parks.

City leagues exist in most cities. The local recreation department will generally be able to inform you as to when and where the leagues will play. Check on the specific requirements, such as liability or health insurance, a physical exam, and/or entry fees.

Summary

1. Volleyball is becoming increasingly popular. The media is increasing its coverage of the game, and players recognize the game as exciting.
2. Beach or sand volleyball is played with two players per side. The rules are somewhat different than the international rules for indoor volleyball.
3. Variations of the game include two-, three-, four-, and six-person teams.
4. Outdoor volleyball strategy must consider the effects of the sun and wind on the way the ball will respond, and how these forces of nature will affect the opponents.

1990-1991 Official Rules United States Volleyball Association*

Rules Differences for 1990-1991

There are no rules changes for the 1990-1991 season. All revisions of the rules are editorial in nature in a continuing effort to make the rule book easier to understand by participants at all levels of competition throughout the United States.

Rule 4, Article 7B: Clarified to indicate that any second penalty issued to the same individual during a game must result in expulsion of the individual for the remainder of the game.

Rule 4, Commentary 1: Defines players and substitutes.

Rule 4, Commentary 8B: Permits coaches to briefly stand near the bench to give instructions to players on the court in a nondisruptive manner. It also permits them to move down the bench to briefly speak to a team member on the bench or warmup area.

Rule 5, Article 1B: The proposed numbering system for jerseys has been eliminated. Numbers may be from 1 thru 99 inclusive.

Rule 5, Current Practices F: Stipulates that if a team does not have numbers of a color sharply contrasting to that of the jersey, the opponents shall be awarded one point at the start of each game.

Rule 6, Article 2: This Article has been reworded to clarify that if the winner of the coin toss elects to serve or receive, the loser has the choice of court to start play. If the winner of the coin toss takes choice of court, the loser may choose to serve or receive.

Rule 7, Article 3: Has been clarified to define the meaning of a term of service. It also clarifies the fact that a serving player may be replaced at any time during playing of the ball. "Hit' is now used for any of the three hits permitted a team to return the ball to the opponents court. Contact of the ball by blockers does not constitute a team hit.

Rule 8, Article 9: This Article has been added to specify the meaning of an attack hit in order to clarify actions described by other Articles.

Rule 8, Article 10: An added Article to specify when a served ball may be legally attacked.

Rule 8, Commentary 8D: The Commentary clarifies that a ball is considered to have crossed the net if it contacts the top of the net and the hands of a blocker above the height of the net. Often times the sound of the ball contacting a blocker's hand through the net will cause confusion when the referee signals a fourth hit by the attacking team after such contact.

---

*Permission granted for reprint by United States Volleyball Association (USVBA). Copyright © 1991.

Rule 8, Commentary 9a: Emphasizes the fact that an illegally attacked ball does not become dead unless it is contacted by the opponents or has completely passed beyond the vertical plane of the net.

The Official Annual USVBA Guide contains information on:
1. Representation to the USVBA Board of Directors, Delegate Assembly, Divisions and Committees, to include the selection/election process
2. Listing of the Player Advisory Council
3. Athlete's Bill of Rights; player and team eligibility rules; grievance and appeal procedures
4. Referee and Scorekeeper certification procedures and Tournament Guidelines
5. Information pertaining to current United States Championships and results from the previous season
6. Awards/Recognition Documentary
7. National and Regional Directory of Leadership and Officials
Regional Leadership and Team Representatives have been issued a copy of the USVBA Guide and may be contacted for information pertaining to the above items. Individuals or Organizations wishing to purchase the USVBA Guide may contact their local USVBA Regional Commissioner or the USVBA Administrative Office, 1750 East Boulder Street, Colorado Springs, CO 80909; phone: (719) 578-4750.

Official Rules 1990-91

Chapter I: Facilities, Playing Area and Equipment

Rule 1 Playing Area and Markings

Article 1. Court—The playing court shall be 18 m long by 9 m wide (59' x 29'6"). A clear area of 2 m (6'6") should surround an indoor court. A clear area of 3 m (9'10") should surround an outdoor court.

Article 2. Court Markings—The court shall be marked by lines 5 cm (2") wide. Areas being defined by court markings shall be measured from the outside edge of the lines defining such area, with the exception of the center line (Article 3).

Article 3. Center Line—A line 5 cm (2") wide shall be drawn across the court beneath the net from sideline to sideline with its axis dividing the court into two equal team areas.

Article 4. Attack Line—In each team area a line 5 cm (2") wide shall be drawn between the sidelines parallel to the center line and 3 m (9'10") from the middle of the center line to the rear-most edge of the attack line. The attack area, limited by the center line and the attack line extends indefinitely beyond the sidelines.

Article 5. Service Area—At a point 20 cm (8″) behind and perpendicular to each end line, two lines, each 15 cm (6″) in length and 5 cm (2″) in width, shall be drawn to mark the service area for each team. One line is an extension of the right sideline and the other is drawn to that its farther edge is 3 m (9′10″) from the extension of the outside edge of the right sideline. The service area shall have a minimum depth of 2 m (6′6″)

Article 6. Overhead Clearance—For all United States Competition, there should be an overhead clearance free from obstruction to a height of 7 m (23′) measured from the playing surface.

Article 7. Substitution Zone—The substitution zone is an area extending from the imaginary extension of the attack line to the imaginary extension of the center line between the court boundary and the scorekeeper's table.

Article 8. Minimum Temperature—The minimum temperature of the playing area shall not be below 10 degrees centigrade (50 degrees fahrenheit).

Commentary on Rule 1—Playing Facilities

1) *Court Clearance—Benches, bleachers, low hanging baskets, or other objects less than 2 m (6′6″) from the court cause the ball to become dead and a replay directed if they interfere with the logical playing of the ball.*

2) *Ceiling Clearance—The ball becomes dead if it contacts the ceiling, or other objects at a height of 7 m (23′) or more above the playing area and a point or side out awarded. A ball contacting the ceiling or other overhead objects between 15′ and 23′ above playable areas shall remain in play. The ball becomes dead if it contacts above the opponent's area or if it contacts above the playing team's area and then falls into the opponent's area (point or side out). Unusually low hanging objects (less than 15 feet above the playable surface) and their supports (vertical or horizontal) shall cause the ball to become dead and a replay directed if they interfere with a logical playing of the ball.*

   a) *Supports for low hanging objects (such as vertical supports for a basketball backboard) are considered as part of the low hanging obstruction. Such support structures below 23′ cause the ball to become dead and a replay directed if they interfere with normal playing of the ball.*

   b) *The ceiling and overhead objects, regardless of height, over nonplayable areas are considered out of bounds and shall cause the ball to become dead. No replay is directed for such contact.*

3) *Service Area—Where the service area is less than 2 m (6′6″) in depth, a line must be taped or painted on the court to provide the minimum clearance during service. After service, the line is ignored.*

   a) *Only the server is permitted to be in the outlined service area until after the ball is contacted for service.*

4) *Other Factors—The playing surface and surrounding areas shall be flat, horizontal and uniform. Play shall not be conducted on any surface that is wet, slippery or constructed of abrasive material.*

   a) *Indoors the playing surface may be natural ground, wood, or of a synthetic material which is smooth and free of any abrasive surface.*

   b) *For outdoor courts, it shall be permitted to have a slope of 5 mm per meter to provide for proper drainage.*

5. *Unsuitable Courts*—*The court, in all cases, must be under the control of the first referee before and during a match. The first referee alone is responsible for deciding whether or not the court is suitable for play. The first referee should declare the court unfit for play when:*
    a) *Play could be dangerous due to any hazardous condition of the court and surrounding area, to include abrasive type surfaces.*
    b) *Improper or defective equipment could be hazardous to players or officials.*
    c) *The court becomes soft or slippery.*
    d) *Fog or darkness makes it impossible to officiate properly.*

6) *Boundary Markers*—*On outdoor courts, wood, metal or other non-yielding materials may not be used since the ground can erode, thus causing lines to protrude above ground level and present a hazard to players. Hollowed out lines are not recommended. The court lines should be clearly marked before the beginning of a match.*
    a) *On an outdoor court, the lines must be clearly marked with whitewash, chalk, or other substance which is not injurious to the eyes or skin. No lime nor caustic material of any kind may be used. Lines must be marked in such a manner as to not make the ground uneven.*
    b) *On indoor courts, the lines must be of a color contrasting to that of the floor. Light colors (white or yellow) are the most visible and are recommended.*

7) *Assumed Extension of Lines*—*All lines on the court, with the exception of the center line, are considered to have an assumed indefinite extension. All rules (with the exception of Rule 9, Article 6) that apply to a zone on the court, apply to like zones outside the court.*

8) *Non-Playable Areas*—*Non-playable areas are defined as:*
    a) *Bleachers or other spectator seating areas*
    b) *Team benches and the area behind team benches*
    c) *Match administration areas and the area behind such areas*
    d) *The area between the scorekeeper's table and team benches*
    e) *Any other area deemed, in the judgement of the first referee, to be unsuitable for normal play or hazardous to the welfare of players and/or officials.*
    Players may not enter non-playable areas for the purpose of playing the ball. Players making a play on the ball may play the ball over non-playable area and may enter a non-playable area after playing the ball if they have at least one foot in contact with the floor at the time the ball is contacted.

10) *Adjacent Courts*—*Where competition (including warm-ups preceding a match) is being conducted on adjacent courts, no player may penetrate into an adjacent court before, during or after playing the ball.*
    a) *Where adjacent courts are in use at the start of a match, the courts shall be considered in use until conclusion of the match.*
    b) *During tournament competition, if a court is scheduled for use, whether the court is occupied or not at the start of a match, the court shall be considered to be in use.*

11) *Dividing Nets or Other Partitions*—*Where dividing nets or other partitions of a movable nature separate adjoining courts, only the player(s) actually making an attempt to play the ball may go into the net or move it. It should be ruled a dead ball and a fault if a teammate, substitute, coach or other person moves the net or partition to assist a play.*

12) *Special Ground Rules*—*Any special ground rules for a match must be specified in the pre-match conference by the first referee.*

13) *Lighting—Lighting in a playing facility should be 500 to 1500 luxes measured at a point 1 m. above the playing surface.*
14) *Scoreboard—No special recommendations are made as to the size of the scoreboard. It should be divided into two parts with large numbers to provide a running score for each team. The name or initials of the two teams should be shown at the top of each side. Information displayed on the scoreboard is not official and may not be used as a basis of protest.*
15) *Bad Weather—In case of bad weather (thunderstorms, showers, high winds, etc.) the first referee can postpone the match or interrupt it as deemed advisable for the protection of all participants.*

Rule 2. The Net

Article 1. Size and Construction—The net shall be not less than 9.50 m. (32') in length and 1 m. (39") in width throughout the full length when stretched. A double thickness of white unmarked canvas or vinyl 5 cm. (2") wide shall be sewn along the full length of the top of the net. The net must be constructed of 10 cm. (4") square dark mesh only. A flexible cable or cord with a minimum breaking strength of 3000 pounds shall be stretched through the top tape and a flexible cable or cord having a minimum breaking strength of 1000 pounds through the lower tape of the net. The ends of the net should be capable of receiving a wooden dowel to keep the ends of the net in straight lines when tight.

Article 2. Net Height—The height of the net measured from the center of the court shall be 2.43 m. (7'11 5/8") for men and 2.24 m. (7'4 1/8") for women. The two ends of the net must be at the same height from the playing surface and cannot exceed the regulation height by more than 2 cm. (3/4").

Article 3. Vertical Tape Markers—Tapes of white material 5 cm (2") wide and 1 m. (39") in length shall be fastened to the net at each end, over and perpendicular to the corresponding side line. The vertical tape markers are considered to be a part of the net.

Article 4. Net Antennas—Coinciding with the outside edge of each vertical tape marker an antenna shall be fastened to the net at a distance of 9 m. (29'6") from each other. The net antennas shall be 1.80 m. (6') in length and made of safe and moderately flexible material with a uniform diameter of 10 mm. (3/8"). The upper half of each antenna shall be marked with alternating white and red or orange bands not less than 10 cm. (4") and not more than 15 cm. (6") in width. The antennas will be affixed to the net with fasteners that provide for quick and easy adjustment for proper alignment. The fasteners shall be smooth surfaced and free of any sharp edges that might be considered hazardous to players.

Article 5. Net Supports—Where possible, the posts, uprights or stands, including their bases, which support the net should be at least 50 cm. (19 1/2") from the sidelines and placed in such a manner as to not interfere with the officials in the performance of their duties.

Commentary on Rule 2—The Net

1) *Net Supports—Net supports should be convenient for referees and should present the least possible hazard for players. They must be of a length that*

allows the net to be fixed at the correct height above the playing surface. Fixing the posts to the floor by means of wire supports should be avoided if possible. If wire supports are necessary, they should be covered with a soft material to provide protection for the players. It is recommended that strips of material be hung from the wire to alert players of their presence.

2) *Net Adjustments—The height and tension of the net must be adjusted before the start of the match and at any other time the first referee deems it advisable. Height measurements should be made in the center of the court and at each end of the net perpendicular to the sidelines to assure that each end of the net is within the prescribed height variation. The net must be tight throughout its length. After being tightened, the net should be checked to assure that a ball striking the net will rebound properly.*

3) *Net Torn During Play—If a net becomes torn during play, other than by a served ball, play shall be stopped and a play-over directed after the net is repaired or replaced. If the net becomes torn by a served ball, a side out will be directed with the opponents serving when play resumes.*

Current Practices for Rule 2

1) Net heights for age groups/scholastic competition—The following net heights are currently in practice for the below indicated age groups and scholastic levels of competition:

Age Groups	Girls	Boys/Coed
18 years and under	2.24 m. (7'4 1/8")	2.43 m. (7'11 5/8")
16 years and under	2.24 m. (7'4 1/8")	2.43 m. (7'11 5/8")
14 years and under	2.24 m. (7'4 1/8")	2.24 m. (7'4 1/8")

Scholastic Levels	Girls	Boys/Coed
Grades 1 thru 6 (Elementary School):		
	1.85 m. (6'1")	1.85 m. (6'1")
Grades 7 thru 9 (Middle School):		
	2.24 m. (7'4 1/8")	2.24 m. (7'4 1/8")
Grades 7 thru 12 (Junior and Senior High School):		
	2.24 m. (7' 4 1/8")	2.43 m. (7'11 5/8")

In the interest of safety for age group and scholastic competition, the height of the net for co-ed play shall be that specified for male competition. This height requirement shall not be modified.

2) USA Youth Volleyball Net Heights—Where competition is being conducted under rules for USA Youth Volleyball, the following net heights are recommended:

Ages 7 thru 9	2.3 m. (7'6 1/2")
Ages 10 thru 12	2.15 m. (7'1")

A higher net height has been recommended for the younger age groups in an effort to have them refrain from attempting to spike the ball and to concentrate on the basics of using three hits to return the ball to the opponents. The lower net height for the older age group will provide an opportunity for them to spike the ball as a natural progression in the overall skills of volleyball.

Rule 3. The Ball

Article 1. Size and Construction—The ball shall be spherical with a laceless leather or leatherlike cover of 12 or more pieces of uniform light color with or without a separate bladder; it shall not be less than 62 cm. nor more than 68 cm. (25" to 27") in circumference; and it shall weigh not less than 260 grams nor more than 280 grams (9 to 10 ozs).

Commentary on Rule 3—The Ball

1) *Approval of Balls—Balls used for sanctioned USVBA competitions must be those approved by the USVBA Committee on Equipment.*
2) *Responsibility for Approval of Match Balls—It is the responsibility of the first referee to examine balls prior to the start of a match to determine that they are official and in proper condition. The first referee shall be the final approving authority for all balls to be used during a match. A ball that becomes wet or slippery during competition must be changed.*
3) *Pressure of the Ball—The pressure of the ball, measured with a special pressure gauge, must be between 0.32 and 0.42 kg/cm2 (4.5 to 6.0 lbs/sq. in.). However, the structure of the ball may affect the maximum variation of the pressure allowed (see manufacturer's marking on the ball); for this reason, the first referee may reduce this margin of difference.*
4) *Markings on the Balls—A maximum of 25% of the total exterior surface area of the ball may be covered with logo, name, identification and other markings and coloring, which is to say that a minimum of 75% of the exterior surface of an approved ball shall be of uniform light color excluding markings.*
5) *Three Ball Retrieval System During a Match—The following procedures will be followed when using the three ball retrieval system during a match:*
   a) *Six (6) ball retrievers will be used and shall be stationed as follows: (1) One at each corner of the court about 4 to 5 m from the end lines and 2 m to 3 m from the sidelines; (2) One behind the scorekeeper (if practical); (3) One behind the first referee.*
   b) *At the start of a match, a ball will be placed on the scorekeeper's table and one given to each of the ball retrievers nearest the serving areas. These retrievers are the only ones authorized to give a ball to the server.*
   c) *When the ball is outside the playing areas, it should be retrieved by one of the ball retrievers and given to the one who has already given a ball to the player making the next serve. If the ball is on the court, the player nearest the ball should immediately place it outside the court.*
   d) *At the instant the ball is ruled dead, the ball retriever nearest the service area will quickly give a ball to the player who will be executing the next service.*
   e) *During a time-out, the first referee may authorize the second referee to give the ball to the retriever nearest the area where the next service will occur.*
   f) *A ball being returned from one ball retriever to another will be rolled, not thrown, along the floor outside the court. A ball being returned should be delivered to the ball retriever who has just given a ball to the server.*

Chapter II: Participants in Competition

Rule 4. Rights and Duties of Players and Team Personnel

Article 1. Rules of the Game—All team members are required to know the rules of the game and abide by them.

Article 2. Team Discipline—The head coach and playing captain are responsible for discipline and proper conduct of team members.

Article 3. Team Spokesperson—The playing captains are the only players who may address the first referee and shall be the spokespersons of their team. The playing captains may address the second referee, but only on matters concerning the second referee's duties. Head coaches may address the referees only for the purpose of requesting a time-out or substitution.

Article 4. Time-Out Requests—Requests for time-out may be made by the head coaches while in the team bench area and/or by the playing captain when the ball is dead.

    a.   Each team is allowed two time-outs in each game. Consecutive time-outs may be requested by either team without a resumption of play between time-outs. The length of a time-out is limited to 30 seconds.

    b.   If a team captain or head coach inadvertently requests a third time-out, it shall be refused and the team charged with an improper request. If, in the judgement of the first referee, a team requests a third time-out as a means of attempting to gain an advantage, the offending team will be sanctioned for a team delay (team yellow card).

    c.   During a time-out, all team members move to the vicinity of the team benches and may participate in discussions. Water and/or other liquids or powders may only be administered in the vicinity of the team bench. Where possible, this area should be at least 2 m (6'6") from the court.

Article 5. Team Benches—Benches or chairs are to be placed on the right and left of the scorekeeper's table not nearer to the center line than the attack line. Team members shall occupy the bench located on the side of the net opposite the first referee adjacent to their playing area. Substitutes are to be seated on their team's bench or be in their team's warmup area.

Article 6. Individual Sanctions—The following acts of team members are subject to sanction by the first referee:

    a.   Addressing officials concerning their decisions.

    b.   Making profane or vulgar acts, gestures or remarks.

    c.   Committing acts or gestures tending to influence officials.

    d.   Disruptive coaching or other actions by any team member.

    e.   Crossing the vertical plane of the net with any part of the body with the purpose of distracting an opponent while the ball is in play.

Article 7. Degree of Individual Sanctions—Offenses committed by team members may result in the following sanctions by the first referee:

    a.   WARNING: For minor unsporting offenses such as talking to opponents, spectators or officials, shouting or other minor unsporting acts that disrupt the conduct of the game, a warning (yellow card) is issued and is recorded on the scoresheet. A second minor offense during the same game by the same team member must result in a penalty (red card).

b. PENALTY: For rude behavior, a second minor offense or other serious offenses, a penalty (red card) is issued by the first referee and is recorded on the scoresheet. A penalty automatically entails the loss of service by the offending team if serving, or if not serving, the awarding of a point to the opponents. A second act warranting the issuing of a penalty to a team member during the same game results in expulsion.

c. EXPULSION: Extremely offensive conduct (such as obscene or insulting words or gestures) towards officials, spectators or other players results in expulsion of a team member from the game (red and yellow cards together) in which the offense occurred. Expelled individuals must leave the court and team area until the next game of the match. A second expulsion during a match must result in the disqualification of the team member(s). No further penalty is assessed.

d. DISQUALIFICATION: A second expulsion during a match, or any feigned, attempted or actual physical aggression towards an official, spectator or opponent results in the disqualification of the team member for the remainder of a match (red and yellow cards held apart). A disqualified team member must leave the area (including spectator area) of the match. No further penalty is assessed.

Article 8. Misconduct Between Games—Any sanctions for misconduct between games will be administered in the game following such misconduct.

Article 9. Improper Team Requests—Any improper request that does not affect play or delay the game shall be denied and noted on the scoresheet. Any additional improper requests during the game shall be sanctioned as a team delay (Article 10). Examples of improper requests are:

a. Requesting a time-out, substitution, lineup check, etc, after the first referee's whistle for service

b. A request for time-out or substitution by other than the head coach or playing captain

c. A second request for substitution during the same dead ball period without an intervening time-out

d. A request for an excess time-out

e. A request for substitution that would result in an excess team or player substitution

f. A request that would result in a wrong position entry

Article 10. Team Delays—A team delay is sanctioned with a warning (yellow card) on the first occasion and a penalty (red card-point or side out) on any subsequent occasion during the same game, regardless of reason. Team delays assessed against a team are indicated by the first referee showing the appropriate signal or penalty card and notifying the coach or playing captain of the reason for the sanction. Such sanctions must be noted in the comments section of the scoresheet. Team delays include:

a. Failure to submit a lineup at least 2 minutes prior to the start of a match or prior to the signal indicating expiration of the intermission between games

b. A second improper request during the same game

c. Delay in completing a substitution

d. A request for entry of an illegal player (not on team roster, disqualified team member, illegal number, etc.)

e. Administering water and/or other liquids near the sideline

f.   Failure to report to the end line when directed to do so at the start of a match and between games of a match

g.   Delay in returning to play after a time-out

h.   Delay in moving to positions for serving or receiving service after completion of a rally

i.   Action by a player which creates an unnecessary delay in the start of play

Commentary on Rule 4—Rights and Duties of Players and Team Personnel

1) *Team Members—Players are defined as the team members on the playing area. Substitutes are team members in uniform who are eligible to enter the game and are located on the team bench or in the warm-up area.*

2) *Conduct Between Games—Any sanction outlined in Articles 6 and 7 may be assessed during the period following the pre-match coin toss and during periods between games of a match. Teams shall be immediately notified when a sanction is imposed against a team member prior to the start of the match or between games of a match. The sanction shall be administered at the beginning of the game following assessment of the sanction. In the case of multiple sanctions, enforcement shall be in the order in which the offenses occur. In the case of simultaneous offenses (such as sanctions assessed against opponents for offenses against each other) the sanction shall be enforced against the serving team first and then against the receiving team. After lineups have been received and recorded on the official scoresheet, sanctions will be recorded by the scorekeeper.*

3) *Conduct During Game—If a team member deliberately performs acts for the purpose of distracting an opponent during play, play shall be stopped and a penalty (individual red card) immediately imposed by the first referee.*

4) *Disqualified Team Members—Disqualified team members will be permitted an opportunity to remain in the vicinity of the bench for a brief period to pick up belongings, etc., provided they refrain from further misconduct. After one minute, if the team member has not departed, the captain shall be warned that further delay will result in a default. If the team member has not departed within 15 seconds after the warning, the game shall be defaulted.*

5) *Disqualification for more than Match—If the first referee feels that a team member has committed a serious unsporting act that warrants disqualification from more than the match in which the act was discovered, or for acts committed between matches, a report must be made to the authorities in charge of the tournament for final action. First referees are authorized to disqualify team members from only the match in which the act occurred.*

6) *Team Benches—Team members shall immediately change benches at the end of each game and when teams change playing areas in the middle of a deciding match.*

   a) *The coach may stand to instruct team members in a nondisruptive manner and may stand and move about to speak to team members provided they do not move closer than one meter from the playing court.*

   b) *A nonplayer team member(s) may sit on the bench or remain in the warmup area during play. The warmup area shall be beyond the team bench nearest the endline of their playing area and not nearer the court than the team bench. No ball may be used for warmup activities except during the period between games of a match.*

(1)   If no warmup area is available for warmup beyond the bench area and away from the court, nonplayer team members must remain on the bench.

c)   *A nonplaying team member guilty of misconduct shall be sanctioned by the first referee. If the team member cannot be identified, the sanction shall be imposed against the head coach, or team member responsible for bench conduct if the head coach is playing in the game.*

7)   *Playing Captain—One of the six players shall be designated as the playing captain. The player designated on the lineup sheet submitted at the start of a game shall remain the playing captain at all times when in the game. When replaced, the playing captain or head coach shall designate another player to assume the duties of playing captain until replaced or the original playing captain returns to the game.*

8)   *Head Coach—One team member on the bench must be designated as the head coach. Should the head coach enter the game as a player, another team member on the bench must be designated as the head coach.*

9)   *Coaching—Non-disruptive coaching is permitted. Acts deemed disruptive by the first referee shall be sanctioned as a major offense without warning. A second such act charged to a nonplayer during a game shall result in that person being expelled. Examples of disruptive acts shall include, but not limited to:*

a)   *Tactics designed to delay the game*

b)   *Loud or abusive language*

c)   *Comments to officials*

d)   *Comments to opposing teams*

e)   *Throwing of objects*

f)   *Displaying disgust in an overt manner*

10)   *Electronic Aids—Electronic devices, such as video recorders, tape recorders, etc., may be used as aids to obtain information for use in post match analyzation. Electronic devices which transmit information from other parts of a facility to the bench area during a match are not considered to be in the spirit of volleyball and shall not be allowed. Discovery of teams using such devices in the bench area shall result in the coach being sanctioned as a major offense (red card) for unsporting conduct and the devices must be removed.*

11)   *Team Sanctions—If a team has been charged with a team delay, any subsequent team sanctions, to include an improper request, must result in a team penalty (team red card).*

12)   *Time-Out Periods—After the first referee's whistle for service, if the second referee blows a whistle in response to a team's request for time-out or substitution, play will be stopped, the team charged with an improper request and a playover directed.*

a)   *Teams granted a legal time-out may terminate the time-out period at any time they indicate they are ready to resume play. If the opponents wish to extend the time-out period, that team shall be required to take a team time-out.*

b)   *If a team fails to return to play immediately upon the signal indicating the end of a time-out period, that team shall be sanctioned for delay (team yellow card).*

    c) *If a team makes a third request for time-out, the request shall be denied and the team charged with an improper request.*

      (1) If the request is inadvertently granted, the time-out shall be terminated immediately upon discovery and the team charged with a team delay (team yellow card).

      (2) If, in the first referee's opinion, the request was made as a means of gaining an advantage, the team shall be sanctioned for a team delay (team red card).

    d) *If team member, other than the head coach or playing captain, requests a time-out, the request will be denied and the team charged with an improper request. If the request results in the granting of a time-out, it shall be terminated immediately and the team sanctioned for delay (team yellow card).*

Rule 5. The Teams

Article 1. Players' Uniforms—The playing uniform shall consist of a jersey, shorts and light and pliable shoes (rubber or leather soles without heels.

a. It is forbidden to wear head gear or jewelry (including taped earrings, string bracelets, etc.), with the exception of medical medallions, religious medallions or flat wedding bands. If worn, medical and religious medallions must be removed from chains and taped or sewn under the uniform. If a ring, other than a flat wedding band, cannot be removed, it must be taped in such a manner as to not create a safety hazard for other personnel. If requested by a team captain or head coach before the match commences, the first referee may grant permission for one or more players to play without shoes.

b. Player's jerseys must be marked with numbers not less than 8 cm (3") in height on the chest and not less than 15 cm (6") in height on the back. Numbers shall be located on the jersey in such a position that they are clearly visible. Numbers shall be in a color clearly contrasting to that of the jersey. (See Current Practice—page 30 of the official rule book.) For United States competition, shirts may be numbered from 1 through 99 inclusive. Duplicate numbers may not be worn.

c. Uniforms [jerseys and shorts (one or two piece), pants or culottes] must be of the same color, style, cut and trim. If t-shirts, boxer shorts, tights, leotards, body suits, bicycle shorts, etc., are worn in such a manner that they are exposed, they will be considered to be a part of the uniform and must be worn by all team members and must be identical. For only one individual to wear any of the above mentioned items, it must be for a verified medical reason. For the purpose of identical uniforms, shoes, socks and knee pads are not considered part of the uniform and are not required to be identical for team members. During cold weather, it is permissible for teams to wear identical training suits provided they are numbered in accordance with the specifications of paragraph b) above and are of the same color, style, cut and trim.

Article 2. Composition of Teams and Substitutions—A team shall consist of six players.

a. Before the start of each match, including during tournament play, teams shall submit a roster listing all team members and the uniform number each player and substitute will wear. Rosters shall also indicate the head coach who must sign the roster. Once the roster has been submitted to the second referee or scorekeeper no changes may be made.

b. At least two minutes before the start of a match and prior to the expiration of the intermission between games, the head coach or team captain shall submit to the scorekeeper or second referee a signed lineup of players in the service order each will play. Lineups will be submitted on the official lineup sheets. After the lineup sheets have been received by the scorekeeper, no changes may be made. Errors in recording lineups on the scoresheet may be corrected if necessitated due to a scorekeeper's error. Players listed on the lineup sheets may be replaced prior to the start of play through a substitution request by the head coach or captain under the provisions of paragraph e) below. One of the players on the lineup sheet must be designated as the playing captain. Prior to the start of play, opponents will not be permitted to see the lineup submitted by the opposing team.

c. Substitutions may be requested by either the playing captain on the court or the head coach when the ball is dead. A team is allowed a maximum of six (6) team substitutions in any one game. Before entering the game, a substitute must report to the second referee in proper playing uniform ready to immediately enter when authorization is given. If the substitution is not completed immediately, the substitution shall be cancelled and the team charged with a delay (team yellow card—Rule 4, Article 10). No additional request may be made until after the next dead ball, or a team has been granted a time-out.

d. The playing captain or head coach requesting a substitution(s) shall indicate the number of substitutions desired and shall report to the second referee the jersey numbers of players involved in the substitution. If the head coach or playing captain fails to indicate that more than one substitution is desired, the first or second referee shall permit only one (1) substitute to enter and charge the team with an improper request. Following a completed substitution, a team may not make a new request for substitution until the next dead ball or until a time-out has been requested and granted to either team. During a legal charged team time-out, any number of requests for substitution may be made by either team. Immediately following a time-out period, an additional request for substitution may be made.

e. Players starting a game may be replaced only once by a substitute and may subsequently enter the game once, but in the original position in the serving order in relation to other players. Only a starting player may replace a substitute during the same game. There may be a maximum of two players participating in any one position in the service order (except in case of accident or injury requiring abnormal substitution under the provisions of paragraph g) below). If an improper substitution request is made (i.e., excess team or player substitution, second request for substitution during the same dead ball period, etc.) the request will be refused and the team charged with an improper request (Rule 4, Article 9). No new request may be made until the next dead ball or one of the teams has been granted a time-out.

f. If a player becomes injured and cannot continue playing within 15 seconds, such player must be replaced or a team time-out is awarded. After that brief period, if the team desires to have the player remain in the game, and if the player cannot continue to play immediately, the team must use a charged time-out. If the player is replaced, regardless of time required to safely remove the player from the court, no time-out shall be charged.

g. If through accident or injury a player is unable to play and substitution cannot be made under the provisions of paragraph e), or if the team has used its allowable six (6) team substitutions, such player may be replaced in the following priority without penalty.

(1) By any substitute who has not participated in the game.

(2) By the player who played in the position of the injured player.

(3) By any substitute, regardless of the the position previously played. Players removed from the game under the abnormal substitution provisions of paragraph g), or substitutes whose injuries create an abnormal substitution due to their inability to enter the game to replace an injured player, will not be permitted to participate in the remainder of the game.

h. If through injury or accident a player is unable to play and substitution cannot be made under the provisions of paragraphs e) and g), the referee may grant a special time-out of up to three (3) minutes. Play will be resumed as soon as the injured player is able to continue. In no case shall the special injury time-out exceed three minutes. At the end of the special time-out, a team may request a normal time-out provided they have not already used their allowable two (2) time-outs. If, after three minutes, or at the expiration of time-outs granted subsequent to the special timeout, the injured player cannot continue to play, the team loses the game by default, keeping any points acquired. No player may be granted more than one (1) three (3) minute injury time-out during any match. If a player becomes injured to the extent that a second (2nd) injury time-out would be required, the match shall be defaulted for the safety of the player.

i. If a team becomes incomplete through expulsion or disqualification of a player, and substitution cannot be made under the provisions of paragraph (e) above, the team loses the game by default, keeping any points acquired.

Article 3. Modified Substitution Rules—For USVBA Senior/Master/ Divisions, USVBA A Divisions or lower, Women's competition governed by NAGWS rules, recreation, senior and junior age group divisions or other levels of competition where the capability of players require more liberal substitution rules to permit teams to be competitive and/or for developmental play, the following modified substitution rules may be used:

a. A team shall be allowed a maximum of twelve (12) substitutions in any one game. A player shall not enter the game for a fourth time (starting shall count as an entry). Players starting a game may be replaced by a substitute and may subsequently re-enter the game twice. Each substitute may enter the game three times. Players re-entering the game must assume the original position in the serving order in relation to other teammates. No change may be made in a player's position in the service order unless necessitated by an injury requiring an abnormal substitution under the provisions of paragraph b) below. Any number of players may enter the game in each position in the service order.

b. If through accident or injury a player is unable to play, and substitution cannot be made under the provisions of paragraph a), or if the team has used its allowable twelve (12) team substitutions, such player may be preplaced in the following priority without penalty:

(1) By the starter or substitute who has played in the position of the injured player, if such starter or substitute has not already been in the game the allowable three times, or by any player who has not already participated in the game.

(2) By any player on the bench who has not been in the game three time, regardless of position previously played.

(3) If all players have been in the game the allowable three times, by a substitute who previously played in the position of the injured player.

(4) By any substitute, even though all substitutes have been in the game the three allowable times.

NOTE: If a substitute is injured to the extent that entry is not possible under the provisions of b) (1) or b) (3), the substitute will not be permitted to participate for the remainder of the game.

c. If through injury or accident a player is unable to play and substitution cannot be made under the provisions of paragraph a) or b), the first referee may grant a special time-out under the provisions of Rule 5, Article 2g).

d. If a team becomes incomplete through disqualification or expulsion of a player and substitution cannot be made under the provisions of paragraph a) above, the team loses the game by default, keeping any points acquired.

Article 4. Wrong Position Entry or Player Illegally in Game—If a player is found to be illegally in the game or playing in a wrong position in the service order, play must be stopped, the player illegally in the game replaced and the following corrective action taken.

a. If the team at fault is serving at the time of discovery of the error, a side out shall be declared and all points scored during that term of service cancelled.

b. If the team at fault is receiving and discovery is after the opponents have served, all points previously scored by the offending team will be retained. The serving team will be awarded a point unless the error is discovered after the serving team has scored a point. In such case, no additional point will be awarded, the illegal player shall be replaced and play continued without further penalty.

c. If it is not possible to determine when the error first occurred, the player(s) wrongfully in the game shall be replaced if the offending team is serving, a side out shall be declared and only the last point in that term of service removed. If the opponent is serving, they shall be awarded a point unless the play immediately preceding discovery of the player illegally in the game resulted in a point.

d. If correction of the error requires a substitution due to an illegal or wrong position entry of a player, neither the team or player(s) will be charged with a substitution. In addition, any player or team substitutions charged at the time of the wrong entry shall be removed from the scoresheet as though they had never occurred.

NOTE: If a substitute is injured to the extent that entry is not possible under the provisions of b) (1) or b) (3), the substitute will not be permitted to participate for the remainder of the game.

Commentary on Rule 5—The Teams

1) *Uniform—Where reference is made to identical uniforms, it is construed to mean jerseys and shorts or a one piece uniform, exposed t-shirts and exposed tights, body suits, bicycle shorts, etc. Reference to home team colors may be ignored where deemed appropriate by match sanctioning authorities.*

2) *Players' and Substitutes' Numbers—Each player and substitute must wear identical numbers on the front and back of the jersey while participating in the game. No player shall participate without a legal number. Players shall wear numbers corresponding with numbers listed for them on team rosters submitted to the scorekeeper prior to the start of a match. Duplicate numbers may not be worn.*

3) *Colors—Numerals must be of a color sharply contrasting to the color of the jersey. Examples of inappropriate combinations would be yellow numerals on white jerseys, navy blue numerals on black jerseys, etc. (See Current Practices—page 171 .)*

4) *Jewelry and Other Articles—If play must be stopped to remove jewelry or illegal equipment, the team shall be sanctioned for team delay (team yellow card). In cases where jewelry cannot be removed, such items must be taped securely.*

   a) *Earrings must be removed. Taping of earrings is not permitted, regardless of reason.*

   b) *Braided hair with beads must be secured so that it will not present a hazard to the player, teammates, or opponents.*

   c) *Wearing a hard cast is prohibited on any part of the body.*

   d) *Wearing hand splints or other type of potentially dangerous protective device on the upper part of the body, arms or hands, or any device that could increase a player's ability to hit the ball in a forceful manner, shall be prohibited, regardless of how padded. The wearing of a soft bandage to cover a wound or protect an injury shall be permitted.*

   e) *The wearing of an "air-filled" type cast on the lower extremities or a protective type knee brace is permissible provided there are no exposed metal or other hard or abrasive parts. A plastic ankle "air-filled cast brace" may be worn provided all plastic parts are fully covered.*

   f) *Prosthetic limbs may be worn provided a medical statement has been obtained and signed by a doctor stating that the limb is no more dangerous to the player or other participants than a corresponding natural limb.*

   g) *"Head gear" is interpreted to mean no hats or bandanas. A sweat band of soft pliable material, or bandana folded and worn as a sweat band, is permissible.*

5) *Required Number of Players—Under no circumstances may a team play with less than six (6) players.*

6) *Substitutions—Only the head coach or the playing captain may ask referees for permission to make a substitution. The head coach must be in the bench area at the time the request is made.*

a)   *Failure to indicate that a multiple player substitution is desired shall limit the team to one substitute. In the event that more than one player attempts to enter, the additional player(s) will be refused entry and the team charged with an improper request (Rule 4, Article 9).*

b)   *After making a request and indicating the number of substitutions desired, if the head coach or playing captain refuses to complete the substitution or reduces the number of substitutions to be made, the team shall be charged with a team delay (Rule 4, Article 10). A new request for substitution may not be made until the next dead ball following assessment of the team delay. EXCEPTION: If a change in request is due to a referee's mind change, the request will be honored and no sanction charged.*

c)   *Substitutes going onto the court must wait by the side of a player illegally in the game, counts as one of the total number of substitutions allowed for the team.*

e)   *Each substitute entering the game, except during replacement of a player found to be illegally in the game, counts as one of the total number of substitutions allowed for the team. A team attempting to make an excess substitution, or players attempting to enter the game an excessive time or in a wrong position in the service order shall cause the team to be sanctioned for an improper request·(Rule 4, Article 9).*

f)   *When either referee notices an injured player, play shall be stopped and a replay directed. If the player indicates that play without replacement might be possible, the first referee may allow the player up to 15 seconds to make such determination. If play is not possible after that brief interruption, the player must be replaced or the team must use a legal time out if the player is to remain in the game.*

   (1)   If removal of an injured player causes a delay, no time-out will be charged, regardless of length of time required to safely remove the player from the court. Safety of the player(s) is the primary consideration.

   (2)   If a substitute is injured to the extent that entry is not possible under the provisions of Article 2,g) (2) to replace an injured player, the substitute will not be permitted to participate in the remainder of the game.

7)   *Submitting Lineups—If a team fails to submit a signed lineup to the scorekeeper or second referee at least two minutes prior to the start of a match or before the signal ending the rest period between games of a match, that team shall be sanctioned for team delay (Rule 4, Article 10). After an additional 15 seconds, if the lineup has not been submitted, the team will be penalized (red card). If the team continues to delay, the first referee shall declare the game a default.*

a)   *Replacement of a player listed on the lineup sheet prior to the start of a game shall count as both a player and team substitution. There is no requirement for a replaced player to participate in a play before being replaced. Such requests shall be governed by the provisions of Article 23), or Article 3a), whichever is appropriate.*

Current Practices for Rule 5

1)   Noncontrasting Color Numbers—If a team does not have numbers of a color clearly contrasting to that of the jerseys, the opponents shall be awarded one point at the start of each game.

Chapter III: Rules of Play

Rule 6. Team Areas, Duration of Matches and Interruptions of Play

Article 1. Number of Games—Matches shall consist of the best two out of three games or the best three out of five games.

Article 2. Choice of Playing Area and Serve—Prior to the start of a match, one team captain will call the toss of a coin. The winner of the toss may elect to serve, receive or take choice of court for the first game.

a.   If the winner chooses to serve or receive, the other team has choice of court.

b.   If the winner takes choice of court, the other team has the choice of serving or receiving first.

Article 3. Choice of Playing Area for Deciding Game—Before the beginning of a deciding game of a match, the first referee makes a new toss of the coin with the options described in Article 2. The team captain not calling the toss of the coin for the first game shall call the toss of the coin for the deciding game.

Article 4. Change of Playing Areas Between Games—After each game of a match, except when a deciding game is required, teams and team members will change playing areas and benches.

Article 5. Change of Playing Area in Deciding Game of Match—When teams are tied in number of games won in a match, and one of the teams reaches eight (8) points (or when four minutes have elapsed in a timed game) in a deciding game, the teams will be directed to change playing areas. After change of areas, serving will continue by the player whose turn it is to serve. In case the change is not made at the proper time, it will take place as soon as it is brought to the attention of the first referee. The score remains unchanged and is not a grounds for protest.

Article 6. Time Between Games of a Match—A maximum interval of three (3) minutes is allowed between games of a match, including the fourth and fifth games of a match. The interval between games includes time required for change of playing areas and submitting of lineups for the next game.

Article 7. Interruptions of Play—As soon as either referee notices an injured player, or a foreign object on the court that could create a hazard or distraction to players, play will be stopped and the first referee will direct a play-over.

Article 8. Interruptions of the Match—If any circumstances, or series of circumstances, prevent completion of a match (such as bad weather, failure of equipment, etc.), the following shall apply:

a.   If the game is resumed on the same court after one or several periods, not exceeding four hours, the results of the interrupted game shall remain the same and the game resumes under the same conditions (same team rosters, officials, score at time of interruption, standings of completed games, etc.) as existed before the interruption.

b.   If the match is resumed on another court or in another facility, results of the interrupted game will be cancelled. The results of any completed game(s) of the match will be counted. The cancelled game shall be played under the same conditions (same rosters, officials, games won and loss standing, etc.) as existed before the interruption.

c.   If the delay exceeds four hours, the match shall be replayed, regardless of where played.

Article 9. Delaying the Game—Any act which, in the judgement of the first referee, unnecessarily delays the game may be sanctioned. (Rule 4, Article 10)

Commentary on Rule 6—
Team Areas, Duration of Matches and Interruptions of Play

1) *Changing Sides—Changing sides during the deciding game of a match must be done with a minimum of delay.*
   a) *Players must assume the same positions they were in before changing playing areas.*
2) *Delaying the Game—In order to clarify the interpretation of Rule 6, Article 9, it is necessary to explain that any attempt to delay the game shall result in a warning from the first referee. If the attempt is repeated, or it is determined that the attempt is deliberate by a player or team, the referee must sanction the player or team by denoting it a serious offense. (Rule 4, Article 10)*

Current Practices for Rule 6

1) One Game Playoff—In a one game playoff, teams shall change sides when one team has scored eight (8) points, or when four (4) minutes have elapsed in timed games. The scoring procedure outlined in Rule 12, Article 2 shall be used for one game playoffs. The "Rally Point" scoring shall not be used.
2) Matches Without Deciding Games—In the interest of consistency, a toss of the coin should be held prior to a third or fifth game of a match in which such games will be played regardless of outcome of preceding games of the match.
   a) In the final game of a three or five game match where all games are played regardless of outcome, teams will change playing areas when one team has scored its eighth point or 4 minutes have elapsed in timed games.
3) Time Game—In circumstances where the efficient management of a tournament or series of matches requires adherence to a time schedule in order to complete the competitions, timed games may be employed. Such timed games may be played on the basis of 8 minutes ball-in-play time or 15 points, whichever occurs first. Such basis must be established before the first game where round robins, a specific number of games, etc., are indicated as the format.
4) Promotional Intermission—If a promotional intermission is to be used, it will be between the second and third games and shall be no longer than 10 minutes in duration, including any warmup time.

Rule 7. Commencement of Play and the Service

Article 1. The Service—The service is the act of putting the ball into play by the player in the right back position who hits the ball with one hand (open or closed) or any part of one arm in an effort to direct the ball into the opponent's area.
   a.   The server shall have five seconds after the first referee's whistle for service in which to release or toss the ball for service.

b. After being clearly released or thrown from the hand(s) of the server, the ball shall be cleanly hit for service. (Exception: If, after releasing or tossing the ball for service, the server allows the ball to fall to the floor without being hit or contacted, the service effort shall be cancelled and a reserve directed. However, the referee will not allow the game to be delayed in this manner more than one time during any term of service).

c. At the instant the ball is contacted for service, the server shall not have any portion of the body in contact with the end line, the court or the floor (ground) outside the lines marking the width of the service area.

d. The service is considered good if the ball passes over the net between the antennas or their indefinite extensions without touching the net or other objects.

e. If the ball is served before the first referee's whistle for service, the serve shall be cancelled and a re-serve directed. A second occasion during the same game by the same player results in a side out.

Article 2. Serving Faults—The first referee will signal side-out and direct a change of service to the other team when one of the following serving faults occur.

a. The ball touches the net.

b. The ball passes under the net.

c. The ball touches an antenna or does not pass over the net completely between the antennas or their indefinite extensions.

d. The ball touches a player of the serving team or any object before entering the opponent's playing area.

e. The ball lands outside the limits of the opponent's playing area.

Article 3. Term of Service—A team continues to serve until it commits a fault. A serving player may be replaced at any time during a term of service.

Article 4. Serving Out of Order—If a team has served out of order, the team loses the service and any points gained while serving out of order if it is discovered before the opponents serve. The players of the team at fault must immediately resume their correct positions on the court.

Article 5. Service in Subsequent Games—The team not serving first in the preceding game of a match shall serve first in the next game of the match, except in a deciding game of a match (Rule 6, Article 3).

Article 6. Change of Service—The team which receives the ball for service shall rotate one position clockwise before serving.

Article 7. Screening—The players of the serving team must not, through screening, prevent the receiving player from watching the server or trajectory of the ball. Screening is illegal and a fault.

a. A team makes a group screen when the server is hidden behind a group of two or more teammates who are standing in an erect position and the ball is served over a member(s) of the group.

b. A player with hands extended clearly above the height of the head or arms extended sideways at service shall be considered to be screening if the ball passes over the player.

Article 8. Positions of Players at Service—At the time the ball is contacted for the serve, the placement of players must conform to the service order recorded on the scoresheet as follows (the server is exempt from this requirement):

a. In the front or back row, the center player may not be as near the right sideline as the right player nor as near the left sideline as the left player. No back row player may be as near the net as the corresponding front row player. After the ball is contacted for the serve, players may move from their respective positions.

b. The serving order, as recorded on the official scoresheet, must remain the same until the game is completed.

c. Before the start of a new game, the serving order may be changed and such changes must be recorded on the scoresheet. It is the responsibility of the head coach or team captain to submit a signed lineup to the scorekeeper prior to the expiration of the authorized rest period between games of a match.

Commentary on Rule 7—Commencement of Play and the Service

1) *The Service—If the server releases or tosses the ball for service, but does not hit it and the ball touches some part of the server's body or uniform as it falls, this counts as an illegal service and the ball shall be given to the other team.*

a) *If the server releases or tosses the ball in a service action and then allows it to fall to the floor without touching it, the first referee shall cancel the serve and direct re-serve for which an additional five seconds is allowed. If the player does not serve within these time limits, the player is penalized by loss of service. Any identical action during the same term of service shall result in an illegal serve and loss of service. Subsequent identical action in the same game by the same player will result in a warning (individual red card) for any additional action by the same player.*

b) *After the whistle for service, no other actions (requests for time-out, lineup check, etc.) may be considered until after the ball has been served, even if the request has been made after a server has initiated service action and legally permitted the ball to fall to the floor. A re-serve is considered to be a part of a single effort to serve and must be completed before any requests may be considered.*

c) *The server is not allowed to delay service after the referee's whistle for service, even if it appears that players on the serving team are in a wrong position or are not ready.*

d) *The server may be standing outside the service area when the first referee blows the readiness to serve whistle, but must be within the legal service area at the time the ball is contacted for service.*

e) *At the moment of service, the server's body may be in the air entirely forward of the end line provided the last contact with the floor (ground) was within the legal service area.*

f) *If a service fault occurs (Rule 7, Article 2) and the opposing team commits a positional fault at the moment of a legal service (Rule 7, Article 8), the serving team scores a point.*

g) *If an illegal service occurs and the opposing team commits a positional fault at the moment of service, the ball is given to the opponents. The service is illegal when:*

(1) *The player serves while in contact with the floor (ground) outside the service area.*

(2) *The ball is thrown or pushed for service.*

(3) *The player serves with two hands or arms.*

(4) *The service is not made following the correct rotation order.*

(5) *The ball is not thrown or released before it is hit for service.*

(6) *Service action is not initiated within five seconds after the first referee's whistle for service.*

2) *Screening—In order for members of the serving team to be called for a group screen at the moment of service, the players must be standing near each other in an erect position and the ball must pass over the area where the players were standing at the moment of contact of the ball for service.*

   a) *If a member of the serving team moves to take a position in front of an opponent near the net after the first referee's whistle for service, the player shall be sanctioned (red card) for unsporting conduct.*

3) *Position of Players—The position of players is judged according to the position of their feet in contact with the floor (ground) at the time the ball is contacted for service. A player who is not in contact with the floor (ground) will be considered to retain the status of the last point of contact with the playing surface. For the purpose of this rule, the service area is not considered to be a part of the court. All players, except the server, must be fully on the court at the time the ball is contacted for service. Players in contact with the center line are governed by the provisions of Rule 9, Article 6. At the instant the server hits the ball for service, all players must be in their proper positions corresponding with the order noted on the scoresheet. A positional fault should be signalled by the referee(s) as soon as the ball has been hit by the server. Occasionally there may be doubt as to whether a player is a front or back row player. In such cases, the referee may delay the whistle and check the scoresheet after play has concluded. If a check of the scoresheet reveals that a player was out of position, the call may be made, even though late.*

4) *Wrong Server—When it is discovered that a wrong player is about to serve the ball, the scorekeeper shall wait until the ball has been contacted for service and then blow a horn/whistle or stop the game in any manner possible and report the fault to one of the referees. Any points scored by the wrong server shall be cancelled, a side-out declared and players of the team at fault must immediately resume their correct positions on the court.*

   a) *If a wrong server is discovered prior to a serve by the opponents, any points scored during that term of service shall be cancelled and a sideout awarded the opponents. Players of the team at fault must assume their correct positions on the court.*

   b) *If discovery of a wrong server is after the opponents have served, all points scored by the wrong server remain legal. The players of the team at fault must assume correct positions on the court and a point is awarded the opponents unless the play immediately preceding discovery of the wrong server resulted in a point. In such case, no additional point is awarded. If discovery is after a sideout by the opponents, the sideout shall be cancelled and the opponents awarded a point.*

Current Practices for Rule 7

1) Preliminary Service Action—Preliminary actions, such as bouncing the ball on the floor or lightly tossing the ball from one hand to the other, shall be allowed, but shall be counted as part of the five seconds allowed for the server to initiate service release or toss of the ball preparatory for the service.

2) Service for Elementary Grade Players—Where elementary grade age players are in a competition, it can be considered legal service if the ball is hit directly from the hand of the server, not necessarily dropped or tossed. Where this serve is acceptable, it should be established in advance or otherwise agreed upon mutually before competition starts and the officials notified. In such levels of team play, players should be encouraged to develop the ability and skills necessary for a serve which does satisfy the requirements of the official rules.

3) Requesting Lineup Check—Team captains may request verification of the service order of their team if done on an infrequent basis. Requests for lineup checks for opponents will be limited to determining whether or not the players are in a correct service order. No information will be provided to disclose which opposing players are front line or back line players.
NOTE: During Junior Olympic age competition, the head coach is also permitted to request a lineup check.

Rule 8. Playing the Ball

Article 1. Maximum of Three Team Hits—Each team is allowed a maximum of three (3) successive hits of the ball in order to return the ball to the opponent's playing area. Blocking does not constitute a team hit.

Article 2. Contacted Ball—A player who contacts that ball, or is contacted by the ball in other than blocking action shall be considered as having played the ball.

Article 3. Contact of Ball with the Body—The ball may contact any part of the body on or above the waist.

Article 4. Simultaneous Contacts with the Body—The ball can contact any number of parts of the body, providing such contacts are simultaneous and that the ball rebounds immediately and clearly after such contact.

Article 5. Successive Contacts—A player may have successive contacts of the ball during blocking (Rule 8, Article 11) and during a single attempt to make the first team hit of a ball coming from the opponents, even if the ball is blocked, provided there is no finger action used during the effort and the ball is not held or thrown. Any other player contacting the ball more than once, with whatever part of the body, without any other player having touched it between these contacts, will be considered as having committed a double fault.

Article 6. Held Ball—When the ball visibly comes to rest momentarily in the hands or arms of a player, it is considered as having been held. The ball must be hit in such a manner that it rebounds clearly after contact with a player. Scooping, lifting, pushing, or allowing the ball to roll on the body shall be considered to be a held ball.

Article 7. Simultaneous Contacts by Opponents—If the ball visibly comes to rest between two opposing players, it is a double fault and the first referee will direct a play-over.

    a.   If the ball is contacted simultaneously by opponents and does not visibly come to rest, play shall continue.

    b.   After simultaneous contact by opponents, the team on whose side the ball falls shall have the right to play the ball three times.

    c.   If, after simultaneous contact by opponents, the ball falls out of bounds, the team on the opposite side shall be deemed as having provided the impetus necessary to cause the ball to be out of bounds.

Article 8. Ball Played by Teammates—When two players of the same team contact the ball simultaneously in other than blocking action (Article 11), this is considered as two team hits and neither of the players may make the next play on the ball.

Article 9. Attack Hit—An attack his is an intentional effort to direct the ball into the opponent's playing area in other than blocking action. A third hit by a team is considered to be an attack hit, regardless of intention. A served ball is not considered to be a attack hit.

    a.   If a player near the net attacks the ball in such a manner that the ball is blocked back into the attacking player, such contact is considered to be first team hit.

Article 10. Attacking the Serve—It is illegal for a player to attack a served ball while the ball is completely above the height of the net. The ball does not become dead until it passes the vertical plane of the net or is contacted by an opponent.

Article 11. Attacking Over Opponent's Playing Area—A player is not allowed to attack the ball on the opponent's side of the net. If the ball is hit above the attacker's side of the net and then the follow through causes the attacker's hand and arm to cross the net without contacting an opponent or the net, such action does not constitute a fault.

Article 12. Assisting a Teammate—No player shall assist a teammate by holding such player while the player is making a play on the ball. It shall be legal for a player to hold a teammate not making a play on the ball in order to prevent a fault.

Article 13. Blocking—Blocking is the action close to the net which intercepts the ball coming from the opponent's side by making contact with the ball before it crosses the net, as it crosses the net or immediately after it has crossed the net. An attempt to block does not constitute a block unless the ball is contacted during the effort. A blocked ball is considered to have crossed the net.

    a.   Blocking may be legally accomplished only by players who are in the front row at the time of service.

    b.   Multiple contacts of the ball by a player(s) participating in a block shall be legal provided it is during one attempt to intercept the ball.
        (1)   Multiple contacts of the ball during a block shall be counted as a single contact, even though the ball may make multiple contacts with one or more players of the block.

    c.   Any player participating in a block shall have the right to make the next contact, such contact counting as the first of the team's three hits.

  d. Back row players may not block or participate in a block, but may play the ball in any other position near or away from the block.

  e. Blocking a served ball is a fault.

  f. Blocking of the ball across the net above the opponent's playing area shall be legal provided that such block is:

   (1) After a player has attacked the ball, or in the first referee's judgement, intentionally directed the ball into the opponent's playing area; or,

   (2) After the opponents have completed their three hits; or

   (3) After the opponents have hit the ball in such a manner that the ball would, in the first referee's judgement, clearly cross the net if not touched by a player, provided no member of the attacking team is in a position to make a legal play on the ball; or

   (4) If the ball is falling near the net and no member of the attacking team could reasonably make a play on the ball.

Article 14. Ball Contacting Top of Net and Block—If the ball touches the top of the net and a player(s) above the net participating in a block and the ball returns to the attacker's side of the net, the attacker's team shall then have the right to three team hits.

Article 15. Back Row Attacker—A back row player returning the ball to the opponent's playing area while forward of the attack line must contact the ball when part of the ball is below the level of the top of the net over the attacking team's area. The restriction does not apply if the back line player jumps from clearly behind the attack line and, after contacting the ball, lands on or in front of the line.

  a. It is a fault when a back line player in the attack zone, contacting the attack line, or its imaginary extension hits the ball while it is completely above the height of the net and causes it to cross completely beyond the plane of the net or intentionally directs the ball towards the opponent's area so that it is contacted by an opponent before fully passing the plane of the net.

Commentary on Rule 8—Playing the Ball

1) Reception of the Ball—Contact with the ball must be brief. When the ball has been hit hard, or during setting action, it sometimes stays very briefly in contact with the hands of the player handling the ball. In such cases, contact that results from playing the ball from below, or a high reception where the ball is received from high in the air, should not necessarily be penalized. The following actions of playing the ball should not be counted as faults:

  a) When the sound is different to that made by a finger tip hit, but the hit is still played simultaneously with both hands and the ball is not held.

  b) When the ball is played with two closed fists on a 2nd or 3rd hit and the contact with the ball is simultaneous.

  c) When the ball contacts an open hand and rolls off the hand backward without being held.

  d) When the ball is played correctly and the player's hands move backwards, either during or after the hit.

  e) When a poorly hit ball is caused to rotate (such as a defective spike where the ball is not hit squarely and is caused to spin, or a set ball that is caused to rotate due to improper but simultaneous contact).

2) *Held Ball on Service Receive—Receiving a served ball with an overhead pass using open hands is not necessarily a fault. Such service receives must be judged the same as any open handed pass. If the served ball is traveling in a low and relatively flat trajectory, receiving it with open hands and passing without holding the ball is extremely difficult. If the serve is high and soft, the pass can be made legally the same as any similar ball crossing the net after service.*

3) *Successive Contacts—A player may have successive contacts with the ball when making the first play on a ball coming from the opponents providing fingers are not used in a passing action to direct the ball. During successive contacts, permitting the ball to roll along any part of the body is illegal and must be called. Direction of the flight of the ball after successive contacts is ignored. Successive contacts on a first received ball must be during one continuous attempt to play the ball.*

4) *Simultaneous Contact Between Opposing Players—The rules are designed to insure the continuity of play. During contact of the ball simultaneously between opposing players, the first referee must not blow the whistle unless the ball is momentarily suspended between the hands of opposing players and clearly comes to rest. In such case, the ball must be replayed without a point or change of service being awarded.*

5) *Simultaneous Contact Between Teammates—When two players on a team attempt to play the ball at the same time, resultant action can cause the appearance of simultaneous contact. Referees must be positive that simultaneous contact has been seen before charging that team with two hits. If there is any doubt, only one hit should be called.*

6) *Spiked Ball—A spiked ball is defined as a ball that is forcibly hit from above the height of the net into the opponent's playing area.*

7) *Blocking—Any ball directed towards the opponent's playing area as an attack hit can be blocked by one or a group of opposing front row players. In order for a player(s) to be considered to be in the act of blocking, some part of the body must be above the height of the net during the effort. Blocking action is terminated when a blocker contacts the floor and has no part of the body above the height of the net.*

   a) *If members of a composite block are to benefit from the rule allowing multiple contacts of the ball by blockers, they must be close to the net and close to each other at the time the ball is contacted by the block. If one member of a composite block is above the height of the net during the effort, all members are considered as having been above the height of the net. If a player is attempting to block, but is separated from the block contacting the ball, contact by the player will count as the first of the team's three hits.*

   b) *Players may take a blocking position with the hands and arms over the net providing there is no contact with the ball until after the opponents have completed an attack hit. Immediately after an attack hit, blockers may contact the ball in an effort to prevent it from crossing the net.*

   c) *Multiple contacts of the ball are legal during blocking action even it can be seen that during the action the ball has contacted in rapid succession:*
      (1) *The hands or arms of one player; or,*
      (2) *The hands or arms of two or more players; or,*
      (3) *The hands or other parts of one or more players on or above their waists.*

d) *If the ball touches the top of the net and the hands of an opposing blocker(s) who is above the net, the ball shall be considered to have crossed the net and been blocked. After such contact, the attacking team is allowed an additional three hits.*

e) *Blockers may reach across the plane of the net outside the antenna, but may not contact the ball over the opponent's playing area is made while any part of the blocker or member of a composite block is outside the antenna across the plane of the net, the block is illegal.*

f) *If a player near the net sets the ball from above the height of the net in such a manner that the ball is blocked back into that player, such contact by that player is considered to be a block.*

8) *Back Row Players—A back row player who is inside the attack zone, or its assumed extension, may play the ball directly into the opponent's playing area if, at the moment of contact, the ball is not completely above the level of the top of the net. If a back row player jumps from the floor clearly behind the attack line, the ball may be spiked or intentionally directed into the opponent's area, regardless of where the player lands after hitting the ball.*

a) *A ball contacted from above the height of the net, and directed towards the opponent's playing area by a back row player on or forward of the attack line, or its imaginary extension, does not become an illegal hit until the ball completely passes beyond the vertical plane of the net or is contacted by the opponents.*

 (1)   If the illegally hit ball is contacted by an opposing back row blocker, it is a double fault and a replay shall be directed.

b) *On a 1st or 2nd team hit, if a back row player on or in front of the attack line contacts the ball from above the height of the net is an attempt to direct the ball to a teammate, the ball remains alive and in play if legally contacted by an opposing player before the ball passes untouched fully beyond the vertical plane of the net. If the ball passes untouched fully beyond the vertical plane of the net, it is a fault.*

c) *Simultaneous contact above the net between a back row attacker and an opposing back row blocker is a double fault.*

d) *If a back row player at the net, along with front row blockers, lifts hands or arms towards the ball in a blocking motion as it comes across the net and is touched by the ball, or the ball touches any of the players in that block, it is a fault; back row players not having the right to participate in a block. However, if the block containing the back row player does not touch the ball, the attempt to block is not considered to be a fault.*

e) *A back row player with part of the body above the net while attempting to play the ball near the net becomes an illegal blocker if the ball is legally attacked or blocked by an opponent into the back row player (including simultaneous contact).*

f) *While back row players may not participate in a block, there is no restriction on their being next to a block for the purpose of playing the ball in other than a blocking action.*

Rule 9. Play at the Net

Article 1. Ball in Net Between Antennas—A ball, other than a served ball, hitting the net between the antennas remains in play. If the ball touches the net after a team's three hits and does not cross the net, the referee should not stop the play until the ball is contacted for the fourth time or has touched the playing surface. (See Rule 10, Commentary 1.)

Article 2. Ball Crossing the Net—To be legal, the ball must cross the net entirely between the antennas or their assumed indefinite extension.

Article 3. Player Contact with Net—If a player contacts the net during play, with any part of the body or uniform, other than hair, it is a fault. If the ball is driven into the net with such force that it causes the net to contact a player, such contact is not a fault.

Article 4. Simultaneous Contact by Opponents—If opponents contact the net simultaneously, it shall constitute a double fault and the first referee shall direct a playover.

Article 5. Contact by Player Outside the Net—If a player accidentally contacts any part of the net supports (e.g. a post, cable, the referee's stand, etc.), such contact shall not be counted as a fault provided that it has no effect on the sequence of play. If the stand, posts, etc., are intentionally grasped or used as a means of support, such action constitutes a fault.

Article 6. Crossing the Center Line—Contacting the opponent's playing area with any part of the body except the feet is a fault. Touching the opponent's playing area with a foot or feet is not a fault providing that some part of the encroaching foot or feet remain on or above the center line.

    a.   It is not a fault to enter the opponent's playing area after the ball has been declared dead.

    b.   It is not a fault to cross the assumed extension of the center line outside the playing area.

        (1)   While across the extension of the center line outside the court, a player of the attacking team may play a ball that has not fully passed beyond the plane of the net. Opponents may not interfere with a player making a play on the ball.

        (2)   A player who has crossed the extension of the center line and is not making a play on the ball may not interfere with an opponent.

Article 7. Ball Penetrating or Crossing the Vertical Plane—A ball penetrating the vertical plane of the net over, below or outside the net, may be returned to a team's side by a player of that team provided the ball has not completely passed beyond the vertical plane of the net when such contact is made. When the ball penetrates the vertical plane of the net, the opponents have an equal right to play the ball.

Commentary on Rule 9—Play at the Net

1)   *Ball Crossing Vertical Plane of the Net—If a ball penetrates the vertical plane of the net over the net, under the net, or outside the antennas, the attacking team is allowed to attempt to play the ball back into their team area. The opponents are not allowed to intentionally touch the ball under the net before the ball passes fully beyond the vertical plane of the net. However, if the ball inadvertently contacts an opponent beyond the plane under the net, the ball becomes dead and is not considered to be a fault by the opponents.*

2)   *Player Contact with Net—Hair contacting the net is not considered a fault.*

3)   *Contact with Opponent's Area—Contacting the opponent's playing area with a hand, or other part of the body other than a foot or feet, is a fault. If a player*

lands on an encroaching foot of an opponent, such contact is ignored unless, in the first referee's judgement, the act is done deliberately to interfere with an opponent.

4) *Contact with Opponent Beyond the Vertical Plane—If a player makes contact with an opponent beyond the vertical plane of the net, and if such contact is inadvertent, the contact shall be ignored. If the contact is intentional, it shall be penalized by the first referee without warning.*

   a) *Flagrant intentional contact shall result in disqualification of the player responsible for the contact.*

Rule 10. Ball in Play/Dead Ball

Article 1. Ball in Play—The ball is considered to be in play when it is legally contacted for service.

Article 2. When Ball Becomes Dead—A ball in play becomes dead when:

a. The ball touches an antenna or the net outside n antenna.
b. The ball does not cross the net completely between the antennas.
c. The ball strikes the floor, floor obstructions or wall.
d. The ball contacts the ceiling or overhead object at a height of 7 m (23') or more above a playable surface or any object above an unplayable area.
e. A player(s) commits a fault.
f. A served ball contacts the net or other object.
g. The first or second referee blows a whistle, even if inadvertently.
h. A player causes the ball to come to rest on a rafter or other overhead object that is less than 7 m above the height of the playing area.
i. The ball contacts an object that is less than 15' above playable surface.
j. The ball passes fully beyond the vertical plane under the net.
k. The ball fully passes beyond the vertical plane of the net outside the antennas.

Commentary on Rule 10—Dead Ball

1) *Inadvertent Whistle—The blowing of an inadvertent whistle causes the ball to become dead immediately. In such cases, the first referee must make a ruling that will not penalize either team. For instance, if the ball has been hit in such a manner that it is falling in an area where no player could logically make a play on the ball, and if the referee blows the whistle before the ball has touched the playing surface, by rule the ball becomes dead immediately. In this case, the first referee should rule as though the ball had touched the playing surface at the time the whistle blew. Another example would be after a third hit with the ball striking the net near the top and the first referee inadvertently blowing the whistle. After the whistle, if the ball were to roll in such a manner that it crossed the net into the defending team's area, the first referee will direct a play over.*

2) *Whistles at Approximately the Same Time—If the second referee blows a whistle in response to a request by a captain or coach at approximately the same time as the first referee blows a whistle for service, play shall be stopped and the first referee shall determine which whistle was blown first. If the whistle of the second referee was blown before, or simultaneously with, the*

whistle for service, the request will be granted. If the whistle of the second referee was after the whistle for service, the request will be denied, an improper request recorded and a new service effort directed.

3) *Ball Contacting Antenna—If the ball contacts the antenna above or below the height of the net, the ball becomes dead.*

Rule 11. Team and Player Faults

Article 1. Double Fault—A double fault occurs when players of opposing teams simultaneously commit faults. In such cases, the first referee will direct a play over.

Article 2. Faults at Approximately the Same Time—If faults by opponents occur at approximately the same time, the first referee shall determine which fault occurred first and shall penalize only that fault. If it cannot be determined which fault occurred first, a double fault shall be declared.

Article 3. Penalty for Committing Faults—The penalty for a team or player committing a fault is:

a. In a non-deciding game, if the serving team, or a player of the serving team commits a fault, a side out shall be declared. If the receiving team, or a player of the receiving team, commits a fault, the serving team shall be awarded a point.

b. In a deciding game, if the serving team, or a player of the serving team, commits a fault, a side out shall be declared and the opponents awarded a point and the ball for service. If the receiving team, or a player of the receiving team, commits a fault, the serving team shall be awarded a point.

Article 4. Team and Player Faults—A fault shall be declared against a team or player when:

a. The ball touches the floor (R10,A2)

b. The ball is held, thrown or pushed (R8,A6)

c. A team hits the ball more than three times consecutively (R8,A1)

d. The ball touches a player below the waist (R8,A3)

e. A player touches the ball twice consecutively (R8,A5) (Exception: R8,A5 and A11)

f. Members of a team are out of position at service (R7,A8)

g. A player touches the net or antenna (R9,A3)

h. A player completely crosses the center line and contacts the opponent's playing area (R9,A6)

i. A player attacks the ball above the opponent's playing area (R8,A9)

j. A back row player while in the attack zone hits the ball while it is entirely above the height of the net into the opponent's playing area (R8,A13)

k. A ball does not cross the net entirely between the antennas (R9,A2)

l. A ball lands outside the court or touches an object outside the court (R10,A1)

m. The ball is played by a player being assisted by a teammate as a means of support (R8,A10)

n. A player reaches under the net and touches the ball or an opponent while the ball is being played by the opponents (R9,C1)

o. Blocking is performed in an illegal manner (R8,A11)
p. A ball is illegally served or a service fault occurs (R7,A2; R7,C1f)

Rule 12. Scoring and Results of the Game

Article 1. When Point is Scored—When a fault is committed by the receiving team, a point is awarded to the serving team.

Article 2. Score of a Non-Deciding Game—A non-deciding game (games 1 and 2 in a best of 3 match and games 1 thru 4 in a best of 5 match) is won when a team scores 15 points and has at least a two point advantage over the opponents. No game shall exceed 17 points. If the teams are tied at 16-16, the first team to score the 17th point shall be the winner.

Article 3. Scoring for Deciding Game—The deciding game of a match shall use the "rally point" system with a point awarded on each service or awarded side out. For example:

a) When a fault is committed by the receiving team, a point is awarded to the serving team

b) When a fault is committed by the serving team, the opponents are awarded a point and the ball for service.

c) When a serving team or serving team player is assessed a penalty, the opponents are awarded a point and the ball for service.

d) The winning score shall be the same as that described in Article 2, above.

e) It is not necessary for the winning team to be serving at the time the winning point is scored.

Article 4. Score of Defaulted Game—If a team does not have sufficient players to start a game, or fails to play after the first referee requests play to begin, that team shall lose the game by default. Score of each defaulted game will be 15-0.

Article 5. Score of Defaulted Game Due to Injury—If a game is defaulted due to a team being reduced to less than six players because of an injury, the defaulting team shall retain any points earned. The winning team shall be credited with at least 15 points or will be awarded sufficient points to reflect a two point advantage over the opponents unless such margin would exceed 17 points.

Article 6. Score of Defaulted Game Due to Expulsion of a Player—If a game is defaulted due to expulsion or disqualification of a player, the defaulting team shall retain any points earned. The offended team shall be credited with at least 15 points or a sufficient number of points to indicate a two point winning advantage over the opponents unless such margin would exceed 17 points.

Article 7. Refusal to Play—If, after receiving a warning from the first referee, a team refuses to play, the entire match is defaulted. The score for each defaulted game is 15-0 and the score of the match is 2-0 or 3-0, depending upon the number of games scheduled for the match.

Article 8. Incomplete Team During Match—If a team is reduced to less than six players and cannot complete the remainder of a match, the opponents shall be awarded sufficient points and games necessary to win the match. The defaulting team keeps points and games won.

Commentary on Rule 12—Scoring and Results of the Game

1) *Scoring for Matches Without Deciding Game—Where scheduling time is a factor, local authorities may find it more practical to use the scoring system outlined in Article 3 (Scoring for Deciding Game) in lieu of Article 2 (Scoring for Non-Deciding Game) for the final game of a match when playing matches consisting of three or five game,s regardless of outcome.*

2) *Insufficient Players to Start—If a team defaults a game due to failure to have sufficient players to start a game at the scheduled time, the score shall be recorded as 15-0. No time-outs may be called by the team until a legal number of players are present to play. An interval of up to 10 minutes shall be allowed for the team to have sufficient players to play the next game. If the team has six players present prior to the expiration of this interval, play shall begin immediately. If, after the 10 minute interval, a team does not have at least six players present and ready to play, the second game shall be declared a default. If the match consists of the best 3 out of 5 games, an additional 10 minute interval shall be allowed before declaring the match a default.*

   a) *If neither team has six players available at match time, each team shall be charged with the loss of one game by default. The next game, if played, would be the third game of the match.*

   b) *Score of each defaulted game is 15-0. Score of a defaulted match is 2-0 or 3-0, depending upon the number of games scheduled to be played.*

3) *Failure to Play—If, during the progress of a game, a team fails to return to play for reasons other than a refusal to play, that team shall be sanctioned for a team delay (yellow card warning). After an additional 15 seconds, if the team still has not returned to play, the team shall be penalized (point or side out). After an additional 15 seconds, if the team still has not returned to play, the game shall be declared a default. The losing team shall retain any points scored and the winning team shall be credited with sufficient points necessary to win the game. A three minute period shall then be granted for teams to change sides of the court and submit lineups for the next game of the match.*

4) *Refusal to Play—After a signal from the first referee, teams shall immediately take their positions on the end line to start a match or game. At the conclusion of an interruption in play, teams shall return to their positions on the court immediately upon the signal of either referee. If a team refuses to do so, they shall be warned by the first referee. If, after the waring, the team still refuses to play, the game and match shall be defaulted. Score of each game will be 15-0 and the score of the match shall be 2-0 or 3-0, depending upon the number of games scheduled to be played.*

5) *Reporting for Match and Game—At the signal indicating the start of a match or the expiration of the interval between games, teams must report immediately to the end line of their playing area.*

   a) *If a team fails to report immediately, that team shall be warned for team delay (yellow card). After 15 seconds, if the team has still failed to report to the end line, the team shall be charged a team penalty (red card). After an additional 15 seconds, if the team has still failed to report to the end line, the game shall be defaulted.*

   b) *A three minute interval shall begin immediately after a game has been declared defaulted by the first referee for unnecessary delay. During the three minute interval, teams shall change sides and submit lineups for the next scheduled game.*

c) *If the same team again fails to report to the end line within the provisions of a) above, the match shall be declared a default by the first referee. A defaulted match shall be recorded as 2-0 or 3-0, depending upon the number of games scheduled.*

6) *Discrepancy in Score—If there is a discrepancy between the scoring section and the running score column of the scoresheet, the scoring section shall be the official score. If there is a discrepancy between the score sheet and the visible scoring device, the scoresheet shall be the official score.*

Rule 13. Decisions and Protests

Article 1. Authority of the Referee—Decisions based on the judgement of the referees or other officials are final and not subject to protest.

Article 2. Interpretation of the Rules—Disagreements with interpretations of the rules must be brought to the attention of the first referee prior to the first service following the play in which the disagreement occurred. The playing captain of the protesting team may be the only one to bring the protest to the attention of the first referee.

Article 3. Appeal of Decision of the Referee—If the explanation of the first referee following a protest lodged by the playing captain is not satisfactory, the playing captain may appeal to the tournament director or Protest Committee. If the protest cannot be resolved, the first referee shall proceed to the scorekeeper's table and shall record, or cause to be recorded, on the scoresheet all pertinent facts of the protest. After the facts of the protest have been recorded, the first referee will continue to direct the game and will forward a report later on the protest in question.

Article 4. Disagreement with the Referee's Decision—If a playing captain disagrees with a first referee's decision in the assessment of a sanction, such decision is not protestable, but the playing captain may state such disagreement in writing on the back of the official scoresheet after completion of the match.

Commentary on Rule 13—Decisions and Protests

1) *Protest Matters not to be Considered—Protests involving the judgement of a referee or other officials will not be given consideration. Some of these items are:*
   a) *Whether or not a player was out of position at the moment of service*
   b) *Whether or not a ball was held or thrown.*
   c) *Whether or not a player's conduct should be penalized.*
   d) *Any other matters involving only the accuracy of an official's judgement.*

2) *Protest Matters to be Considered—Matters that shall be received and considered by the first referee concern:*
   a) *Misinterpretation of a playing rule.*
   b) *Failure of the first referee to apply the correct rule to a given situation.*
   c) *Failure to impose the correct penalty for a given violation.*

3) *Recording Facts—The following facts should be recorded on the scoresheet concerning any protest situation:*
   a) *Score of the game at the time of the protest.*
   b) *All players in the game at the time of the protest and their positions on the court.*

c) *Player substitutions and team substitutions made prior to the protested situation.*

d) *Team time-outs charged prior to the protested situation.*

e) *A synopsis of the situation that caused the protest to be lodged, the rule violated or omitted, or the penalty improperly imposed.*

f) *Signatures of the scorekeeper, both captains and the first referee to indicate that the facts have been correctly recorded.*

4) *Protest Committee Action—Where possible in tournament play, it is advisable to have a protest committee assigned and available to rule upon a protest situation as soon as possible, preferably prior to the first service following the protest. Such action will preclude having to play the match over from the point of protest if the protest is upheld. The situation can be immediately corrected and only the play in question played over.*

5) *Protest Ruling and Effect—After considering the facts of the protest, the ruling authority may rule that the protest was valid and should be upheld or that the protest was not valid and should be denied. If the protest is upheld, the game will be replayed from the moment in the game immediately preceding the play which prompted the lodging of a protest. If the protest is denied, the score and situation will remain as though the protest had never been lodged.*

6) *Disagreement with Referee's Decision—If a playing captain disagrees with a sanction imposed by the first referee, such disagreement may be expressed on the scoresheet by the playing captain after the conclusion of the match. The playing captain is not allowed to express complaints about decision pertaining to ball handling, or other similar judgement situations pertaining to the playing of the ball on the scoresheet.*

Chapter IV: Officials and Their Duties

NOTE: Chapter IV is included as a guideline for officials and shall not be construed to be a part of the official playing rules subject to protest by team.

Questions regarding techniques and mechanics of officiating should be referred to: Techniques and Mechanics of Officiating: Jim Stewart, Chairman, and Wink Davenport, Chairman, USVBA/FIVB International Arbitres and Neill Luebke, U.S. National Rules Interpreter.

Rule 14 The First Referee

Article 1. Authority of the First Referee—The first referee is in full control of the match and any judgement decisions rendered by the first referee are final. The first referee has authority over all players and officials from the coin toss prior to the first game of a match until the conclusion of the match, to include any periods during which the match may be temporarily interrupted, for whatever reason.

Article 2. Questions not Covered by Rule—The first referee has the power to settle all questions, including those not specifically covered in the rules.

Article 3. Power to Overrule—The first referee has the power to overrule decisions of other officials when, in the first referee's opinion, they have made errors.

Article 4. Position of First Referee During Match—The first referee shall be located at one end of the net in a position that will allow a clear view of the play. The referee's head should be approximately 50 cm. (19 1/2") above the top of the net.

Article 5. Imposing Sanctions—In accordance with Rule 4, the first referee sanctions violations made by players and other team members.

Article 6. Use of Signals—Immediately after blowing the whistle to stop play, the first referee shall indicate by use of hand signals the nature of the fault and the result of the play (point, sideout, playover, etc.).

Commentary on Rule 14—The First Referee

1) *Signaling Service—The first referee will blow a whistle at the beginning of each play to indicate that service shall begin and at any other time judged to be necessary.*

2) *Interrupting Play—Each action is considered finished when the first referee blows a whistle, other than to initiate service. The first referee should only interrupt play when certain that a fault has been committed, and should not blow the whistle if there is any doubt.*

3) *Time-Outs—When teams have returned to the playing area after a time-out, the first referee signals the number of time-outs that have been taken by each team.*

4) *Requesting Assistance—Should the first referee need to deal with anything outside the limits of the court, the first referee should request assistance from the event organizer and/or team members.*

5) *Overruling Officials—If the first referee is certain that one of the other officials has made an incorrect decision, the first referee has the power to overrule that official and apply the correct decision. If the first referee feels that one of the other officials is not correctly fulfilling duties outlined by the Rules, the referee may have the official replaced.*

6) *Suspending the Match—Should an interruption occur, particularly if spectators should invade the court, the referee must suspend the match and ask organizers and the captain of the home team to re-establish order within a set period of time. If the interruption continues beyond that period of time, or if one of the teams refuses to continue playing, the first referee must instruct all officials to leave the playing area. The first referee must record the incident on the scoresheet and forward a report to the proper authority within 24 hours.*

7) *Authority of the First Referee—Although the first referee is in full control of the match and any judgement decisions rendered are considered final, this in no way relieves the right of the playing captains to protest and record matters allowed under the provisions of Rule 13, Article 3.*

Rule 15. The Second Referee

Article 1. Position During Match—The second referee shall take a position on the side of the court opposite and facing the first referee.

Article 2. Assisting the First Referee—The second referee shall assist the first referee by making calls such as:

a. Faults of the center line and attack line.

b. Contact with the net by a player.

    c.   Contact of the ball with an antenna or not crossing the net entirely inside the antenna on the second referee's side of the court.

    d.   Foreign objects entering the court and presenting a hazard to the safety of the players.

    e.   Faults by back row attacker/blocker.

    f.   Performance of duties in addition to those outlined when instructed to do so by the first referee.

Article 3. Keeping Official Time—The second referee shall be responsible for keeping official time of time-outs, warmups, and intervals between games of a match.

Article 4. Conduct of Participants—The second referee shall supervise the conduct of team members on the bench and shall call to the attention of the first referee any unsporting actions of players or other team members.

Article 5. Supervision of Substitutions—The second referee shall authorize substitutions requested by playing captains or the head coach of the teams.

Article 6. Service Order of Teams—The second referee shall verify at the beginning of each game that players of both teams are in positions corresponding with the lineups submitted to the scorekeeper. The second referee shall supervise the rotation and positions of the receiving team players at the time of service.

Article 7. Giving Opinions—The second referee shall give opinions on all matters when requested to do so by the first referee.

Article 8. Ending Play—Play is considered as ended whenever the second referee blows a whistle.

Commentary on Rule 15—The Second Referee

1) *Reporting Time-Outs—When a team takes a time-out, the second referee signals to the first referee the number of time-outs that each team has taken. When the teams return to the court after the conclusion of a time-out, the second referee shall signal the number of time-outs each team has taken.*

2) *Substitutions—The second referee will authorize a substitution when the substitute is ready to enter the game. Before allowing the substitute to enter the court, the second referee will make certain that the scorekeeper has the necessary information to properly record the substitution.*

3) *Control of the Ball—The second referee shall be responsible for assuring that the game ball is at the scorekeeper's table or in the position of a line judge during interruptions of play.*

4) *Replacing First Referee—Should the first referee be suddenly indisposed, it shall be the responsibility of the second referee to assume the duties of first referee.*

5) *Assisting First Referee—The second referee will make calls and perform duties in addition to those outlined when instructed to do so by the first referee.*

6) *Verifying Lineups—When teams change playing areas during the middle of a deciding game of match, it is the duty of the second referee to verify that players are in their correct service order as listed on the scoresheet if requested to do so by a playing captain or head coach.*

7) *Giving Information to Team Captains—Upon request of a playing captain for verification that the opponents have the correct server or that the opposing players are in the game legally, the first referee may direct the second referee that the players are correct or incorrect. No direct identification of opposing*

players positions be limited to infrequent occasions. If it is found that the players are in an incorrect position or illegally in the game, the first referee will direct the second referee and scorekeeper to correct the error.

Rule 16. The Scorekeeper

Article 1. Position During Match—The scorekeeper's position is on the side of the court opposite the first referee and behind the second referee.

Article 2. Recording Information—Prior to the start of a match, the scorekeeper will clearly print the names of the 1st referee, 2nd referee and scorekeeper on the scoresheet. The scorekeeper will obtain and verify team rosters for the match. The scorekeeper will obtain lineup sheets from the teams and record the jersey numbers of starting players on the scoresheet. Once a lineup or team roster has been submitted to the scorekeeper, no changes may be made. Between games of the match, the scorekeeper reminds the second referee to obtain new lineups from captains or coaches in order to properly record changes in lineups. In addition, the scorekeeper:

a. records the scores as the match progresses.

b. makes sure that the serving order and rotation of players is followed correctly.

c. carefully checks eligibility of substitutes before authorizing their entry into a game.

d. records substitution information on the scoresheet.

e. records time-outs taken by teams and notifies the referees of the number of time-outs which have been charged to each team.

Article 3. During Deciding Game of Match—During the deciding game of a match the scorekeeper signals the referees when one of the teams has scored an eighth point and indicates that the teams should change playing areas.

Article 4. Verification of Final Score—At the conclusion of a game, the scorekeeper verifies the final results of the game by signing the appropriate block of the scoresheet.

Commentary on Rule 16—The Scorekeeper

1) *Giving Information to Teams—The scorekeeper, when requested to do so by one of the referees, must tell either of the head coaches or playing captains the number of substitutions and/or time-outs that have been charged to their team. Information pertaining to opponents will not be given to a head coach or playing captain by the scorekeeper.*

2) *Lineups—Prior to the start of each game of a match, the head coach or team captain must submit a signed lineup to the scorekeeper or second referee on the official form provided. Prior to the start of play, opponents will not be permitted to see the lineup of players submitted by the opposing team.*

3) *Recording of Remarks—The scorekeeper must record all remarks pertaining to sanctions, protests, etc., that occur during the progress of the game.*

4) *Order of Service—The scorekeeper must control the order of service. If a wrong server is in the service position at the time the first referee whistles for service, the scorekeeper shall wait until the ball is contacted during service and then sound a horn/whistle and notify the referees of the fault.*

5) *The Score—The scorekeeper must record each point made by a team. The scorekeeper must make sure that the score on the visible scoreboard agrees with the score recorded on the scoresheet. In the event of a discrepancy, the scoresheet shall be official and the discrepancy is not a grounds for protest by a team.*

6) *Final Result of Games—Results of games are final and official when the scoresheet is signed by the scorekeeper.*

Rule 17. The Line Judges

Article 1. Position During Match—During the match, the line judges will be stationed.

a   With two line judges, they must be placed diagonally opposite from each other, one at each end of the court at the corner away from the service area near the intersection of the end line and side boundary line.

b.   With four line judges, one line judge shall be placed opposite each service area with the sideline extended approximately 2 m behind the end line. One line judge shall be placed approximately 2 m outside the sideline nearest the service area in line with the end line extended. Each line judge watches the line to which assigned.

Article 2. Duties—Line judges shall signal the first referee when a:

a.   Ball lands inbounds (signal 3 or signal 2)

b.   Ball lands out of bounds (signal 5 or signal 4)

c.   Foot fault occurs by server or other player (signal 8 or signal 2)

d.   Ball touches, passes over or outside an antenna (signal 8 or signal 4)

e.   "Pancake save" ball touches the floor during an attempted save (signal 2 or 3)

f.   Ball contacts player before going out of bounds (signal 7 or signal 6)

g.   Ball contacts an overhead object (signal 25)

Article 3. Signal Flags—The use of signal flags by line judges shall be at the discretion of the first referee.

Commentary on Rule 17—The Line Judges

1) *Position During Match—During the match, line judges shall be standing in their assigned areas and shall move from those areas only for the purpose of avoiding interfering with players playing the ball or to better observe a ball crossing the net near an antenna.*

2) *Number of Line Judges—For important competitions, it is recommended that four line judges be used.*

3) *Signaling the First Referee—Whenever a line judge needs to attract the attention of the first referee due to a fault committed by a player, or to a rude remark made by a player, the flag or hands shall be raised above the head and waved from side to side.*

Game Procedures

1.   **Officials**

a)   The officials should be certified referees and scorekeepers of the United States Volleyball Association.

2. **Uniforms**
   a) All players must wear uniforms prescribed by USVBA rule 5.
   b) All non-playing referees must wear the official uniform described in Section 4 of the USVBA Guide.

3. **Pre-Game Procedures**
   a) Well ahead of starting time for the first game of a match, the first referee will call team captains together and conduct a coin toss.
   b) After the coin toss, the first referee will supervise warm-up periods with the serving team having use of the court for the first three minute warm-up period if the captains have elected to use separate warm-ups. If the team captains elect to warm-up together on the court, the first referee shall allow six minutes.
   NOTE: In the event that a team does not choose to use its time on the court, the court shall remain unoccupied.
   c) At the end of the warm-up period, the first or second referee will walk to the center of the court and blow a whistle to indicate that the warm-up period is over and players are to clear the court.
   d) Referees and other officials take their places.
   e) Teams line up on the end line of their respective areas. When both teams are ready and facing each other, the first referee will blow a whistle and motion for teams to take their positions on the court.
   f) Second referee will verify that players are on the court in positions listed on the official lineup sheets submitted to the scorekeeper by each team. No corrections may be made unless there has been an error or omission made by the scorekeeper or unless a legal substitution has been made prior to the start of play under the provisions of Rule 5, Commentary 7b. No other changes may be made in the lineups to correct an error made by teams in preparing the lineup sheets.

4. **Start of the Game**
   a) As soon as lineups are verified and teams are ready, the whistle is blown and visual sign is given by the first referee for service to begin.
   b) Prior to the serve, offensive players will halt their movements to allow officials to determine their positions. Continual movement may be misconstrued as screening.

5. **Substitution Procedures**
   a) Substitutes should approach the second referee in the substitution zone and wait to be recognized for entry. Substitutes entering the court and players leaving the court shall touch hands in the substitution zone and wait to be authorized to enter by the second referee.

6. **End of Game and Start of Next Game**
   a) Following the blowing of a whistle indicating the end of a game, players should line up on the end line of their playing areas. When both teams are in position and the second referee has verified that the winning point has been recorded, the first referee will blow a whistle and dismiss the teams for the rest period between games. players may then leave the court.
   b) At the end of the rest period, the second referee will blow a whistle and teams shall immediately report to the end of their playing areas for the next game.

7. **Change of Playing Areas During Game**
   a) When teams are required to change playing areas during a deciding game of a match, the first referee will blow a whistle and indicate both teams to move to the end line of their respective playing area.
   b) After both teams are in position, the first referee will blow a whistle and motion for both teams to proceed in a counter-clockwise direction to the opposite end without delay.
   c) Substitutes and other team personnel will change benches so as to be seated adjacent to their playing area.
   d) When teams are in position on the end line of the new playing areas, the first referee will blow a whistle and motion for both teams to move onto the court.
   c) The second referee will then verify that players are in their correct positions on the court.

8. **At the End of the Match**
   a) Following the whistle indicating the end of a match, players will line up on the end line of their respective playing areas.
   b) When both teams are in position and the second referee has verified that the winning point has been recorded by the scorer, the first referee will blow a whistle and motion for teams to form a single line and proceed to the center of the court to shake hands with opponents.
   c) The second referee will assure that the game ball is returned to the designated area for safekeeping.
   d) Referees will then immediately depart the area of the court.

Commentary on Game Procedures

1) *Substitutes Entering Game—Substitutes entering the game shall wait in the substitution zone until authorized to enter by the second referee. If a player enters without authorization, the player shall be directed to return to the substitution zone and the team warned by the first referee. While there is no intent to make protocol a major part of the game, failure of a player(s) to follow proper procedures can cause errors in the recording of information by scorers.*

2) *Verification of Scoresheets—At the conclusion of each game, the second referee will check with the scorer to assure that a winning score has been attained and will then notify the first referee. The scorer will then verify the final official score of the game by signing the scoresheet in the appropriate block on the scoresheet.*

OFFICIAL NCAA VOLLEYBALL BOX SCORE FORM

Site: _____ Date: _____ Attendance: _____

TEAM:			ATTACK				SET			SERVE		PASS	DEF	BLOCK		
NO	PLAYER	GP	K	E	TA	PCT.	A	TA	PCT.	SA	SE	RE	DIG	BS	BA	BE
TEAM TOTALS																

TEAM ATTACK PER GAME   TOTAL TEAM BLOCKS

	Game 1				
	2				
	3				
	4				
	5				

GAME SCORES	1	2	3	4	5	TEAM RECORDS

TEAM:			ATTACK				SET			SERVE		PASS	DEF	BLOCK		
NO	PLAYER	GP	K	E	TA	PCT.	A	TA	PCT.	SA	SE	RE	DIG	BS	BA	BE
TEAM TOTALS																

TEAM ATTACK PER GAME   TOTAL TEAM BLOCKS

	Game 1
	2
	3
	4
	5

KEY
GP = Games Played
K = Kills
E = Errors
TA = Total Attempts
PCT = %
KILL PCT = (K − E) + TA

A = Assists
  (Servers Only)
ASSIST PCT = A + TA
SA = Service Aces
SE = Sevice Error
RE = Reception Errors

D = Digs
BS = Block Solos
BA = Block Assists
BE = Block Errors
Team Blocks = BS + ½BA
Individual Blocks = BS + BA

Length of Match _____   1st Referee _____

2nd Referee _____

UNITED STATES VOLLEYBALL ASSOCIATION

VOLLEYBALL

SCORE SHEET

TOURNEY

PLACE

DIVISION

COURT   MATCH

Date   Day

Time match scheduled

Time game started

Time game finished

TEAM

SERVING ORDER	PLAYERS NUMBERS	SCORE AT TIME OF SUBSTITUTION		
1				
2				
3				
4				
5				
6				

SCORE

first   serve

SERVING ORDER   SCORE

1   1   1
2   2   2
3   3   3
4   4   4
5   5   5
6   6   6
7   7   7
8   8   8
9   9   9
10 10 10
11 11 11
12 12 12
13 13 13
14 14 14
15 15 15
16 16 16
17 17 17
18 18 18
19 19 19
20 20 20

TEAM

SERVING ORDER	PLAYERS NUMBERS	SCORE AT TIME OF SUBSTITUTION		
1				
2				
3				
4				
5				
6				

time outs

SUBSTITUTIONS   1 2 3 4 5 6

SUBSTITUTIONS   1 2 3 4 5 6

COMMENTS:

Code

Served ◯   Point ③   Rotate Ⓡ   Play over Ⓟ   No serve ☐   Mind change M

Score of Game   1 2 3 4 5   pts.

WINNING TEAM

LOSING TEAM

SIGNATURES

NAME

referee

umpire

umpire

UNITED STATES VOLLEYBALL ASSOCIATION

VOLLEYBALL
SCORE SHEET

TOURNEY

PLACE

DIVISION

COURT ____ MATCH

Date 2/2/90 Day FRIDAY

Time match scheduled

Time game started

Time game finished

X first serve

TEAM: PENN STATE

SERVING ORDER	PLAYERS NUMBERS	SCORE AT TIME OF SUBSTITUTION			
1	5		(R)(R)(R)		
2	3		(1)(2)(3)(R)(R)		
3	4		(4)(R)(R)(6)(7)(R)		
4	16		(R)(R)(R)(8)(R)		
5	8	5-9	(6)(R)(R)		
6	2	5-9	(R)(R)		

SCORE:
(1)(2)(3)(4)(5)(6)(7)(8)(9)(10)(11)(12)(13)(14)(15) 16 17 18 19 20
(1)(2)(3)(4)(5)(6)(7)(8) 9 10 11 12 13 14 15 16 17 18 19 20

time outs
5-6 0-3
8-12

SUBSTITUTIONS 1 F 3 4 5 6

COMMENTS:

TEAM: PEPPERDINE

SERVING ORDER	PLAYERS NUMBERS	SCORE AT TIME OF SUBSTITUTION			
1	14		(R)(3)(4)(5)(6)(R)		
2	15		(1)(R)(2)(R)		
3	7		(R)(8)(9)(R)(10)(R)		
4	10		(2)(R)(R)		
5	13		(R)(R)(11)(12)(13)(R)(15)		
6	1		(R)(R)		

SUBSTITUTIONS 1 2 3 4 5 6

Code
Served ◯	Point ③	Rotate (R)	Play over (P)	No serve ☐	Mind change M

Score of Game ①2 3 4 5   pts.

	NAME		SIGNATURES
WINNING TEAM	PEPPERDINE		15
LOSING TEAM	PENN STATE		8

referee BILL MADARA

umpire SCOTT ATKINSON

umpire KRISTY PAWLING

USA MEN'S VOLLEYBALL TEAM STATISTICAL SUMMARY

Game	ATTACK K-E / Atts.	Att. Eff.	Kill %	E/B	BACK ROW K-E / Atts.	%	SERVE Pts. / Atts.	Ave.	A/E	Pts. / Atts.	RECEIVE Ave.	(PP) %	E	1	2	C	F	BLOCK	POINTS +	−
1												( ) %								
2												( ) %								
3												( ) %								
4												( ) %								
5												( ) %								
Match Total												( ) %								
Opponent Hitting Errors _____						Opponent _____			Opponent _____										

	Serve	Hitting	Blocking	Opponent Attack Errors	Other Errors		Total
USA	_____	_____	_____	_____	_____	=	_____
Opponent	_____	_____	_____	_____	_____	=	_____

#	ATTACK K-E / Atts.	Att. Eff.	Kill %	E/B	BACK ROW K-E / Atts.	%	SERVE Pts. / Atts.	Ave.	A/E	Pts. / Atts.	RECEIVE Ave.	(PP) %	E	1	2	C	F	BLOCK	POINTS +	−
1												( ) %								
2												( ) %								
3												( ) %								
4												( ) %								
5												( ) %								
6												( ) %								
7												( ) %								
9												( ) %								
10												( ) %								
12												( ) %								
13												( ) %								
15												( ) %								

Official Outdoor Rules*

1.0 Basic Rules

1.1   Teams are composed of two players. Other popular formats utilize three, four, or six persons per team. These guidelines deal chiefly with two-person competition.

1.2   No substitutions may be made after the first serve of the first match. If one player cannot continue play for any reason, his/her team must forfeit.

1.3   A team must keep the ball from contacting the playing area of its court.

1.4   A team may contact the ball no more than three times, and must send the ball over the net and into contact with either an opponent or his court.

1.5   If the serving team sends over a ball that is not returned or lands in the opponent's court, a "point" is awarded.

1.6   Should the team who receives the serve win the rally, a "sideout" is awarded. They receive no point, but become the serving team for the next play.

1.7   Most tournaments utilize a double elimination format in which a team continues to compete until it has lost two matches. Teams with one loss complete against other teams with one loss in the "Losers' Bracket." A team must win any game by at least two points.

1.7a   All matches (winners and losers) on the Pro Beach tour are one game to 15 points. It is the sole prerogative of the tournament director to change the format if tournament conditions, in his opinion, warrant: (i.e., losers' games played to 11 points because of limited daylight.)

1.8   The tournament director organizes and supervises the tournament. Generally, he/she collects an entry fee from players to offset expenses. He/she possesses the authority to make all decisions pertaining to entries, seeding, starting times and rule interpretation.

1.8*   The AVP (Association of Volleyball Professionals) is responsible for determining the scoring method to be used for each event, and will also provide the system to determine seeding for each event.

2.0 Court and Equipment

2.1   The court is a 60 foot by 30 foot rectangle enclosed by, and including, boundary ropes or other means of marking.

2.2   The net is extended between two vertical uprights (poles) at a height of 8 feet for men, or 7 feet, 4 inches of women. The net should be 3 feet

---

*Reprinted with permission by Association of Volleyball Professionals (AVP). Copyright © 1991.

high from top to bottom, and 30 to 32 feet in length when stretched. A cable or strong rope runs through the upper seam of the net. All ropes, cables, and netting are considered part of the "net," and are alive during play. The ball is in play after touching the net.

2.3   The pole (upright) and fixtures attached to the pole are part of the "pole." Should a ball contact the pole during play, the ball is dead.

2.4   The ball should be spherical with a minimum of 12, and a maximum of 18 panels. It should not be less than 26 inches, or more than 28 inches in circumference. Any ball provided by the tournament director may be used. He/she determines the brand and the model. The players will agree on a particular ball of the brand and model. If players cannot decide on a ball within their designated warm-up time, it is the referee's prerogative to decide on the ball to be used. The game ball may be replaced during the game, provided all players agree, or if the referee determines the ball has been damaged to the point that it noticeably affects play; (i.e., noticeable loss of air pressure or a torn panel).

2.4*   The AVP will determine the brand and model of volleyball to be used for each AVP-sanctioned event and must provide a sufficient number of balls for the competition.

3.0 Officials

3.1   The referee is preferably positioned at either end of the net, with his/her eyes two to three feet above the net, so he has a clear view of both sides of the court. Otherwise, he/she should station himself/herself beneath the net.

3.2   The referee makes decisions on all matters not specifically covered in the rules. When the referee is undecided concerning a rule, the head official will make the final determination. Lacking a head official, the tournament director will make the final determination.

3.3   The referee decides if a violation occurred, a ball contact is legal when the ball is dead, when a point has been made, when there is a net violation, and his judgement of the facts is final.

3.4   Should the referee judge that he has made a call by mistake, thereby interrupting play, the point is replayed.

3.5   Players are encouraged to call their own contacts with the net or a mis-handled ball. They are to also call "lines," i.e., in or out about the perimeter of the court. The referee, however, has responsibility for calling and making final decisions regarding the play.

3.6   When the ball is dead, players may ask the referee for explanations regarding play.

3.7   A referee may be replaced by the tournament director or by unanimous agreement of the players. A paid referee may only be replaced by the head official or, if not available, the tournament director. Players may request the head official or tournament director to observe a referee's performance.

3.8   The referee can grant a "time-out" to a player only when the ball is dead. Two time-outs of one minute duration are allowed per team in each game. Time-outs may be taken consecutively without any play in between.

3.9   The referee will stop play when a foreign object enters the court, including a ball from another court. In all such cases, the point will be replayed.

3.10   A player may call a "ball on" only if the ball is on, or has been on the court during play. If a player is playing on a bannered court, the ball must be within, or have been within the banners. A player stops play at his own risk if another foreign object enters the court. In such cases the referee will rule.

3.11   The referee will stop play should a player sustain an injury. If an injury occurs during play, play continues until the ball is dead. Maximum time-out for injury will be at the sole discretion of the head official or, lacking a head official, the tournament director.

3.12   The referee declares when play is to commence.

3.13   Play continues until a violation or time-out is called by the referee, or until the ball touches the ground, the pole, or an object outside the court.

3.14   If a violation occurs after the ball has hit the ground, but during the normal course of "continuation" of the play, the violation will be called by the referee; (i.e., a player hits a ball which contacts the opposing team's court after which his forward momentum carries him into the net.) The referee will determine when the play has ended.

3.15   There cannot be successive violations on the same play after the referee calls a violation, all subsequent play is dead.

3.16   Players will be asked to officiate. If they fail to officiate, they will be penalized. In first round matches, the top seeded teams (as many as necessary), will be responsible for officiating. After the first round, a member of the losing team in the previous round will referee the next round.

3.17* Players refusing to take their turn refereeing may be forfeited out of the tournament or subsequent tournaments and required to pay a fine. Tardiness for a match will also result in a fine.

4.0 Service

4.1   To commence play, the referee will toss a coin. The team winning the toss may select either choice of sides or first service.

4.2   Teams will switch sides of the court every five points in a game to 15 points, and every four points in a game to 11 points.

4.3   The ball may be served from any point behind and between the endlines.

4.4   The server may not step on or touch the endline in any way, or contact the playing surface until the ball is contacted. He may not perceptibly move the endline forward during service, thereby reducing the size of the playing area. However, he may break the imaginary plane above the endline as long as he has contacted the ball before he touches the playing surface. Violation will result in a sideout.

4.5   The server must contact the ball with his hands, fists, or arms.

4.6   The serve must pass over the net between the poles, and touch either an opponent's body or the opponent's court. (Boundary lines are part of the court.)

4.7   A ball may not contact the net on service. Whether a ball contacted the net on the serve is the sole determination of the referee.

4.8   The teammate of the server must be within the court in a motionless position at the time of the serve.

4.9   The teammate of the server may not obstruct the view, intentionally or unintentionally, of the players receiving the serve. At their request, he must move to grant them a clear view of the server's action.

4.10   The server must serve when directed to do so by the referee. If he does not comply, the serve may be awarded to the other team.

4.11   Teammates are to alternate the serve each time their team earns a sideout. It is the responsibility of any team to make sure the opposing team is serving in order.

4.12   There is no penalty for serving out of order.

4.13   An incorrect server, once he has initiated his serve (contact of the ball) will be allowed to complete the duration of his service.

4.14   If a player has served out of order, the opposing team will stay in their original order of service, but the offending team will reverse their original order of service to insure that no player will serve three consecutive times.

4.15   A player continues to serve until the opposition scores a sideout.

4.16   A team may only score a point when it has served the ball.

4.17   If the receiving team is not ready and makes no attempt to play the ball, the play goes over. The referee decides in cases of dispute.

5.0 Ball Contact

5.1   The ball may be contacted with any part of the body.

5.2   The ball may be contacted no more than three times by a team.

5.3   A player may not contact the ball twice in succession, with the exception of "driven balls," and contact while blocking. (See 5.10 and 6.11.)

5.4   After the third team contact, the ball must cross over the net between the poles and land in the opponent's court, or touch an opposing player.

5.5   If the ball contacts any part of the pole, it is a foul.

5.6   If, after three contacts, any part of the ball passes over the pole, it is a foul. The ball must pass entirely within the poles or its extensions.

5.7   A ball that contacts the net, or ropes and cables within the poles that support the net, is legal and in play. (Exception—Service)

5.8   The ball may be played anywhere on or off the court, but may not pass over the net more than once during a team possession.

5.9   The ball must be cleanly hit. If, in the judgement of the referee, the ball comes visibly to rest during contact, the contact is illegal. A legal is one continuous motion. The ball cannot come to rest in the setter's hands.

5.10   A "hard driven" ball may be contacted multiple times in succession by a player if these contacts occur during one effort to play the ball. This counts as one team contact. A "hard driven" ball may never be allowed to come to rest or "carried."

5.11   A ball that is "hard driven" by a block back into the attacking team's court may be contacted multiple times in succession by a player if these contacts occur during one attempt to play the ball.

5.12   If both players on a team contact a ball simultaneously, it counts as one team contact only.

5.13 If the ball contacts the ground and a player simultaneously, the ball is dead.

6.0 Net Play

6.1 A player may not contact the net with any part of his body or clothing. The referee is responsible for calling and making final decisions on these plays. It is not a violation if a player is wearing a hat and the hat contacts the net after inadvertently falling off the player's head.

6.2 If the force of the ball carries the net into contact with a player, there is no violation.

6.3 A ball (other than the serve) that contacts the net is still in play.

6.4 If any part of the ball contacts the pole or passes over a vertical extension of the pole, it is out of play.

6.5 A player may cross under the vertical plane of the net if he does not interfere with the opponent's play. Interference, which results in a point or side-out to the opposing team, is not determined by physical contact but by whether or not, in the referee's opinion, the offended player's ability to make a play was infringed upon.

6.6 No player may interfere, or threaten to interfere, with an opponent's play.

6.7 Any player may attempt to defend his court by blocking the ball as it crosses the net. A player is determined to be blocking when he is positioned within arm's distance of the net with his hand above his shoulder.

6.8 A blocker can block **any ball** crossing the vertical plane of the net, whether the opposing team contacts the ball at the net or not.

6.9 A blocker can contact the ball multiple times, as long as it is judged by the referee to be one attempt. This then, constitutes the team's first contact only.

6.10 A blocker who has made the first team contact in a single effort to block the ball can then make the second team contact.

6.11 Any player may block a ball on the opponent's side of the court when the attacking team has completed its attack. A team is deemed to have completed his attack when:

a. The attacking team has made their third contact of the ball

b. Any time the attacking team has, in the referee's opinion, intentionally directed the ball into opponent's court

c. Any time the attacking team has made an unsuccessful attempt to attack the ball (i.e., a swing and a miss)

6.12 The blocker may not block over the net on a first or second contact by the attacking team unless, in the referee's opinion, the attacking team intentionally directed the ball into the opponent's court.

6.13 If the opposing team has not completed its attack, the blocker may not first contact the ball on the opposing team's side of the net. Simultaneous contact by the blocker and attacker is legal.

6.14 A blocked ball may be directed by the blocker but may not come to rest or "carried" by the blocker.

6.15 If two opposing players contact the ball simultaneously above the net, and the ball comes visibly to rest in their mutual contact, a replay is declared by the official.

6.16   A player may accidentally contact the pole during the play, but not in such a way that it gives him an advantage in making the play.

7.0 Setting

7.1   Rotation shall not be an automatic determination of a violation.

7.2   The ball may not come visibly to rest in setter's hand.

7.3   The ball must be contacted simultaneously by both hands during the set.

7.4   A ball need not travel in the same direction the setter is facing; however, the setter cannot hold or carry the ball to change the direction of the set.

7.5   When the ball is intentionally "set" into the opponent's court, the player must be "squared up" or perpendicular to the line of flight of the ball when setting the ball.

8.0 Player Conduct

8.1   The referee shall have the power to impose a fine to any player who commits, in the referee's opinion, any of the following gross violations of sportsmanship:
a. Persistently addresses the official in regard to decisions.
b. Makes derogatory remarks about, or to, an official.
c. Commits acts derogatory to the official or tending to influence their decisions or deceive them.
d. Makes personal and derogatory remarks about or to opponents.
e. Use of profanity.
f. Any other conduct considered unsportsmanlike.

8.2   A fine will be assessed against a player each time he intentionally kicks or hits the ball out of the area of play before, during or after a match.

8.3   Any player intentionally damaging any of the equipment (nets, balls, poles, ropes, etc.), will be assessed a fine, and be required to pay for the damaged equipment.

8.4   A player shall not commit any act which, in the opinion of the referee, tends to slow down the game unnecessarily. When the referee indicates readiness to play, the server shall not delay, but shall then immediately initiate the serve.

8.5*   Any player who signs up for a tournament, but fails to show up for that event, will be subject to a fine and forfeited out of a subsequent tournament(s).

8.6*   Physical assault of any referee, tournament official, or any other tournament participant by any player, shall result in immediate disqualification from participation in any sanctioned tournament of the AVP for a period of one year. In extreme instances (major injury), a player may be disqualified for life.

9.0 General Tournament Policy

9.1   The tournament director is the final judge on all issues pertaining to when and where games are to be played. He also ensures that courts are safe and playable.

9.2   The head official, or lacking a head official, the tournament director is responsible for providing a referee for each match. Assignment of referees to courts will be their sole prerogative. Usually a member of the losing team on a given court will referee the subsequent game on that court. Players refusing to take their turn refereeing may be forfeited out of the tournament or subsequent tournaments.

9.3   Players shall be responsible for finding the starting time of all their matches and appearing on time. When a match is called up, each team has 15 minutes to warm-up. After this time has expired, the match must begin. Players may be fined and/or assessed points for tardiness. The tournament director must provide starting time information upon request.

9.4   Disputed rule interpretations may be appealed to the tournament director who must have a written copy of the rules at the tournament.

9.5   In the event of a double finals, there will be a three (3) minute rest period provided between games.

9.6   Any unusual formats or rule modifications governing a specific tournament should be expressed in writing and circulate to all players prior to the start of the tournament.

10.0 How to Run a Tournament

10.1   The tournament board is customarily drawn the night before a tournament. The two basic criteria for seeding tournaments are: 1) computer rankings, and 2) player ratings. When all the teams in the tournament have been rated, they may be written on the tournament board. The numbers to the left of the bracket board indicate the seeding positions.

10.2   On the morning of the tournament, it is best to "work the board" from top to bottom so both spectators and players can follow the order of play.

10.3   Tournaments can be run in a variety of formats including double elimination, single elimination, ad round robin play.

10.4   Double elimination seems to be the most preferable, using a "Winners' Bracket" for undefeated teams, and a "Losers' Bracket" for once-defeated teams. Play progresses until two teams are left: one undefeated (winner of the Winners' Bracket), and the once-defeated team (winner of the Losers' Bracket). The final match proceeds with the once-defeated team needing two victories to win the tournament.

16 Team Tournament—Double Elimination

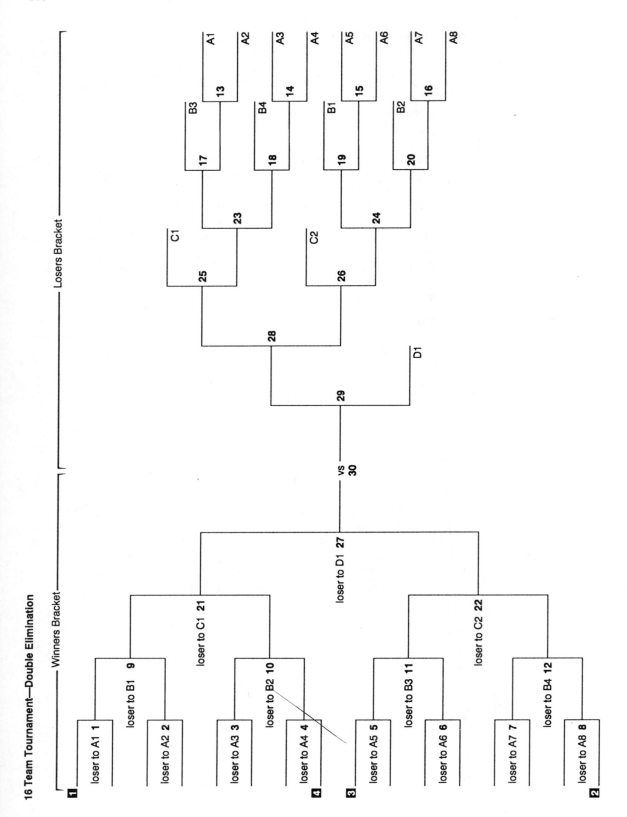

AVP Pro Beach Volleyball Tour Guidelines

In addition to the Rules published in the AVP Rule Book the following guidelines should be followed.

11.0 Setting

11.1 The following are suggestions for faster play, better spectator information, and better tournament efficiency:

11.2 Tournament sign-up. Player must sign up for each event by 5:00 p.m. the Wednesday prior to any tournament. (Sign-ups may be made by phone, mail or in person). Late sign-ups will result in a penalty fee determined by the competition director.

Entry fees and tournament registration. All entry fees must be paid and all entry forms must be completed by 8:45 a.m. Saturday. Late registration and entry fee payment will result in a penalty fee determined by the competition director..

11.3 Starting times. Matches should begin at 9:00 a.m. on Saturday morning. Losers' Bracket games on Sunday morning should begin at 8:00 a.m. Winners' Bracket games should begin at 9:00 a.m. To help ensure prompt starting times, tournament directors should provide four losers' bracket courts and two winners' bracket courts on Sunday morning.

11.4 Warm-up times. Teams will have fifteen (15) minutes to warm-up after match is announced by tournament director.

11.5 Delay of game. Players may not noticeably delay the game. When referee signals to continue play, the match must continue. If not, fines may be assessed. Additionally, a player may not leave the court without calling a time-out.

11.6 Referees. Paid referees should be supplied on both Saturday and Sunday. Referees will be responsible for calling all mishandled balls, nets and player touches. Referees should have whistles, watches and red and yellow cards.

11.7 Sand and sweat. Towels and towel-ball boys should be provided for all Sunday afternoon matches.

11.8 Water breaks. Water breaks may only be taken during side switches.

11.9 Spectator information. A rotating scoreboard with scorekeeper should be situated above the crowd in clear view of the spectators.

The referee should be seated above the volleyball pole in clear view of the spectators. Êhe referee should make visual hand signals to indicate fouls and points.

Tournament announcer should keep crowd well informed by introducing each player on the court, announcing each player's individual sponsor, announcing some previous high finishes and past accomplishments, and keeping the spectators consistently updated on the match score.

When players are introduced on the PA, they should raise a hand so spectators know who is being introduced.

12.0 Individual Player Sponsor Guidelines

12.1　Player identification. All tournament participants should wear swimming trunks, t-shirts, tank tops and sweat shirts with first initial and complete last name printed in clear visible letters on the back.

13.0 Incomplete Tournament Play

13.1　The following is a list of guidelines to use when contemplating whether or not to continue tournament play because of questionable weather conditions.

13.2　Playing conditions.

a. Safety is first and foremost.

b. Quality of play is second. (Not as much emphasis should be placed on this condition).

*The competition director will make decisions on both these conditions. The competition director will also make the final decision on whether or not to continue the tournament.

13.3　Discontinued tournament.

a. Completed match. A match will be judged complete when a team has scored 10 points or more and is ahead by 2 points or more.

b. Prize money distribution.

Teams will be awarded prize money according to their respective record after the last complete round of competition.

Example: The tournament is cancelled before all the games in a certain round are completed. The games which were completed in this round become null and all of the teams in this round receive equal status.

Teams with no losses after the last complete round of competition is finished will equally divide either all or the first portion of prize money. Teams with one loss will receive no prize money or the second portion of prize money.

Example: If the tournament is cancelled before semifinals of the winners' bracket is played, then the four teams in the winners' bracket will equally divide first through fourth place and the eight teams in the losers' bracket will equally divide fifth through ninth place.

c. Tournament title. No team may claim title to any tournament that is not complete.

13.4　Accelerated tournament policy. The competition director will have the power to establish an accelerated tournament policy where games may be shorted in an effort to finish the tournament.

13.5　Player options. If the competition director selects to continue tournament play with questionable weather conditions, individual players may decide to play or not to play and prize money should be distributed accordingly.

13.6　Tournaments with no player participation or limited participation where the first round of competition is not completed. Teams will be awarded prize money according to their respective seed in the tournament, with first seed receiving first place prize money and so on down the line.

14.0 Site Playing Condition Guidelines

14.1 The following is a list of guidelines that a site upon inspection should provide.

14.2 Playing area. The playing area should be of a level nature with neither a noticeable upslope or downslope nor an undulated, hilly or rolling appearance.

14.3 Sand quality.

a. The sand should be of a fine and non-abrasive quality which is not injurious to the skin upon repeated contact.

b. The sand should be loose and easily penetrated to a depth of 7". Beyond a depth of 7" the sand can be of a firmer or more packed nature, but not solid or rock-like.

c. The sand should be free of foreign objects including wood, rocks, glass and metal.

d. The sand should be of such a quality that normal play will not result in excessive and offensive dust in the air for either the players or spectators.

14.4 Playing area parameters. The playing area should be large enough for a minimum of 4 courts, but more appropriately 7 courts. This would constitute a minimum area of 200' x 90' if 4 courts were laid side by side and a minimum of 315' x 60' if 4 courts were laid end to end.

14.5 Surrounding area measurements.

a. There should be sufficient area surrounding the playing courts to accommodate all the equipment (stage, tents, etc.) synonymous with an A.V.P. event.

b. There should be sufficient area surrounding the playing courts to comfortably accommodate the spectators.

14.6 General site specifications.

a. A site should be readily accessible to staff, players, and spectators.

b. A site should provide adequate parking for staff, players, and spectators.

International Champions

Men's International Competition

Olympics

1964 Tokyo
1. USSR
2. Czechoslovakia
3. Japan
USA finished 9th

1968 Mexico City
1. USSR
2. Japan
3. Czechoslovakia
USA finished 7th

1972 Munich
1. Japan
2. East Germany
3. USSR
USA did not compete

1976 Montreal
1. Poland

2. USSR
3. Cuba
USA did not compete

1980 Moscow
1. USSR
2. Bulgaria
3. Rumania
USA did not compete

1984 Los Angeles
1. USA
2. Brazil
3. Italy

1988 Seoul
1. USA
2. USSR
3. Argentina

World Championships

1949 Czechoslovakia
1. USSR
2. Czechoslovakia
3. Bulgaria
4. Rumania
5. Poland
USA did not compete

1952 USSR
1. USSR
2. Czechoslovakia
3. Bulgaria
4. Rumania
5. Hungary
USA did not compete

1956 France
1. USSR
2. Czechoslovakia
3. Rumania
4. Poland
5. Brazil
USA finished 7th

1962 USSR
1. USSR
2. Czechoslovakia
3. Rumania
4. Bulgaria
5. Japan
USA did not compete

1966 Czechoslovakia
1. Czechoslovakia
2. Rumania
3. USSR
4. East Germany
5. Japan
USA finished 11th

1970 Bulgaria
1. East Germany
2. Bulgaria
3. Japan
4. Czechoslovakia
5. Poland
USA finished 18th

1974 Mexico City
1. Poland
2. USSR
3. Japan
4. East Germany
5. Czechoslovakia
USA finished 14th

1978 Italy
1. USSR
2. Italy
3. Cuba
4. Korea
5. Czechoslovakia
USA finished 19th

1982 Argentina
1. USSR
2. Brazil
3. Argentina
4. Japan
5. Bulgaria
USA finished 13th

1986 France
1. USA
2. USSR
3. Bulgaria
4. Brazil
5. Cuba

Women's International Competition

Olympics

1964 Tokyo
1. Japan
2. USSR
3. Poland
USA finished 5th

1968 Mexico City
1. USSR
2. Japan
3. Poland
USA finished 8th

1972 Munich
1. USSR
2. Japan
3. Korea
USA did not compete

1976 Montreal
1. Japan

2. USSR
3. Korea
USA did not compete

1980 Moscow
1. USSR
2. East Germany
3. Bulgaria
USA did not compete

1984 Los Angeles
1. China
2. USA
3. Japan

1988 Seoul
1. USSR
2. Peru
3. China
USA finished 7th

World Championships

1952 USSR
1. USSR
2. Poland
3. Czechoslovakia
4. Bulgaria
5. Rumania
USA did not compete

1956 France
1. USSR
2. Rumania
3. Poland
4. Czechoslovakia
5. Bulgaria
USA finished 9th

1960 USSR
1. USSR
2. Japan
3. Czechoslovakia
4. Poland
5. Brazil
USA finished 6th

1962 USSR
1. Japan
2. USSR
3. Poland
4. Rumania
5. Czechoslovakia
USA did not compete

1966 Czechoslovakia
1. Japan
2. USA
3. Korea
4. Peru

1970 Bulgaria
1. USSR
2. Japan
3. Korea
4. Hungary
5. Czechoslovakia
USA finished 11th

1974 Mexico City
1. Japan
2. USSR
3. Korea
4. East Germany
5. Rumania
USA finished 12th

1978 USSR
1. Cuba
2. Japan
3. USSR
4. Korea
5. USA

1982 Peru
1. China
2. Peru
3. USA
4. Japan
5. Cuba

1986 Czechoslovakia
1. China
2. Cuba
3. Peru
4. East Germany
5. Brazil
USA finished 10th

Men's International Competition
World Cup

1965 Poland
1. USSR
2. Poland
3. Czechoslovakia
USA did not compete

1969 Germany
1. East Germany
2. Japan
3. USSR
USA did not compete

1973 Czechoslovakia
1. USSR
2. Poland
3. Czechoslovakia
USA finished 6th

1977 Japan
1. USSR
2. Poland
3. Cuba
USA finished 10th

1981 Japan
1. USSR
2. Cuba
3. Brazil
USA did not compete

1985 Japan
1. USA
2. USSR
3. Czechoslovakia

1989 Japan
1. Cuba
2. Italy
3. USSR
USA finished 4th

Women's International Competition
World Cup

1973 USSR
1. USSR
2. Japan
3. Korea
USA finished 6th

1977 Japan
1. Japan
2. Cuba
3. Korea
USA finished 10th

1981 Japan
1. China
2. Japan
3. USSR
USA finished 4th

1985 Japan
1. China
2. Cuba
3. USSR
USA did not compete

1989 Japan
1. Cuba
2. USSR
3. China
USA did not compete

Championship Results

Team Championship Results

Year	Champion	Year	Champion
1970	UCLA	1981	UCLA
1971	UCLA	1982	UCLA
1972	UCLA	1983	UCLA
1973	San Diego State	1984	UCLA
1974	UCLA	1985	Pepperdine
1975	UCLA	1986	Pepperdine
1976	UCLA	1987	UCLA
1977	Southern Cal	1988	USC
1978	Pepperdine	1989	UCLA
1979	UCLA	1990	USC
1980	Southern Cal		

Team (Years Participated)

Army (1973)
Ball State (1970-71-72-73-74-79-84-85)
George Mason (1984-85)
Long Beach St. (1970-73)
Ohio State (1975-76-77-78-80-81-82-83-86)
Penn State (1981-82-83-86)
Pepperdine (1976-77-78-83-84-85-86)
Rutgers-Neward (1977-78-79-80)
San Diego State (1972-73)
Southern Cal (1977-79-80-81-82-85-86)
Springfield (1971-74-76)
UC Santa Barbara (1970-71-72-74-75)
UCLA (1970-71-72-74-75-76-78-79-80-81-82-83-84-84-89)
Yale (1975)

Volleyball Resource Directory

Each of these organizations devotes full-time staff attention to the development of volleyball programming that can impact your career, teams, and programs. If you have questions or need assistance, contact these groups and take advantage of the resources they have in their offices.

> United States Volleyball Association
> 3595 E. Fountain Blvd.
> Colorado Springs, CO 80910-1740
> Tel: (719) 637-8300
> Fax: (719) 597-6307

The National Governing Body for the sport in the U.S. Concerned with development of the sport at levels—from youth and Junior Olympic to adult, coed, and national team participation, coaching education, officiating, and more.

> American Volleyball Coaches Association
> 122 2nd Ave., Suite 201
> San Mateo, CA 94401
> Tel: (415) 375-8113
> Fax: (415) 342-7828

An association committed to the development and advancement of volleyball throughout the nation. The Association has unified coaches at every level by increasing the professionalism of its members. The official AVCA Journal, *Coaching Volleyball* and the newsletter, *American Volleyball*, keep coaches abreast of volleyball techniques and activities.

> Volleyball Festival Network
> 4200 Montruse Blvd., Suite 430
> Houston, TX 77004
> Tel: (713) 524-0767

An alliance of school, club and collegiate women's volleyball programs devoted to promoting women's volleyball through research, training and developmental events.

Resources

The USVBA, and its CAP program, offer valuable coaching resources, including new books, videos, action wear, and much more. Call 1-800-638-1502 to obtain a catalog and any texts or other items.

Coaching Volleyball Successfully
The CAP Level I textbook (Included with Level I course registration).

CAP Annual Manual
1st ed. (1988) Articles by CAP Cadre

USA CADRE Collection
2nd ed. Articles by CAP Cadre

1991 IMPACT Manual
Fundamental ethics, drill creation, resources, history and more.

1991 Collegiate Recruiting Guide Book
For players and coaches.

Sport Quotes for Coaches
4th ed. Hundreds of volleyball specific motivational quotes.

Strength Training & Conditioning for VB
A CAP Level II textbook (included with Level II course registration).

Beginning Volleyball Programs
3rd ed. How to start a coach in a youth program.

Junior Olympic Program Guide
3rd ed. How to start, manage, and promote a J.O. program.

1991 Case Book
Officiating examples for USVBA competition.

Sport for a Lifetime Video
Youth volleyball, basic skill techniques.

AVCA Volleyball Handbook
Theories and philosophies of 18 top coaches.

Lion's Cup Video
All Japan Elementary School Championship.

JO Highlight Video
USA Age Group Championship Excerpts.

Volleyball Game Theory and Drills
350 Techniques and Team Drills

Index